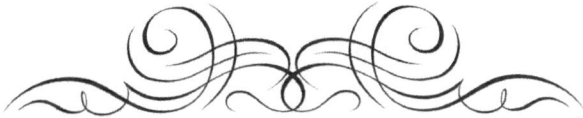

YOU'VE GOT THIS!

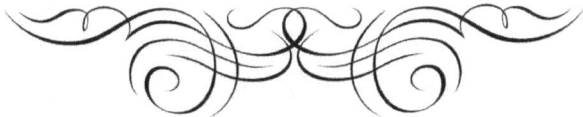

DALE BARR

YOU'VE GOT THIS!

© 2013 Dale Barr

Cover art © Dale Barr

ISBN-13: 978-0-9899486-0-9

ISBN-10: 0989948609

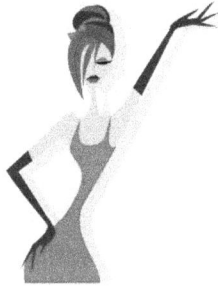

DEDICATION

First and foremost, this book is dedicated to everyone out there who has struggled to maintain a healthy weight or who finds themselves routinely engaged in mental combat with food and exercise. Life is not meant to be lived in constant battle! May this book teach you that food and exercise are tools to use in weight management but that the real secret to sustainable weight loss comes from within. Once you get your Mind in the game, you'll be surprised to find that keeping off unwanted pounds and leading a healthy lifestyle is much easier (and more fun!) than the war you've been waging against yourself, your pantry and your gym membership.

This book is also dedicated to my parents, who left me their legacy of unwavering tenacity and the conviction that anything really worth doing takes persistence and stubborn determination. As my dad told me time and time again, "When there's a will, there's a way."

Contents

INTRODUCTION   1

DAY 1: You're On Your Way!   14

DAY 2: Culinary Panic Attacks   20

DAY 3: The Value of Timeouts   28

DAY 4: What Superhero Are You?   33

DAY 5: Let's Have a Party! (A Pity Party, That Is….)
38

DAY 6: Permission to Fail   44

DAY 7: Can I Get a Little Persistence?   50

DAY 8: Complacency   54

DAY 9: Patience Is a Virtue…Just Not One of Mine
60

DAY 10: The Tortoise and the Hare   67

DAY 11: Acceptance and Surrender   72

DAY 12: Discipline vs. Willpower   77

DAY 13: Cancel-Clear!   82

DAY 14: It's All About the Swag!   86

DAY 15: Tapping Into Your Intuition   89

DAY 16: Sometimes It's Just a Matter of Science   94

DAY 17: Help! I'm Being Sabotaged!   99

DAY 18: The Importance of Packaging   105

DAY 19: In Defense of Setting Boundaries and Acting
With a Healthy Dose of Selfishness   111

DAY 20: Breaking It Down   117

DAY 21: Expecting vs. Believing   121

DAY 22: Slow Progress Is Better Than No Progress
128

DAY 23: Holy Smokes! I Really HAVE Established
New Habits!   132

DAY 24: Resistance, Acceptance, Change   135

DAY 25: It's an Invitation, Not an Obligation…Nor a
Death Sentence!   140

DAY 26: The Answer Is Never in the Refrigerator   146

DAY 27: Failure vs. Setback   150

DAY 28: The Power of Words   155

DAY 29: Relapse Prevention Planning   160

DAY 30: Setting Other Goals   164

INTRODUCTION

First, a Little About Me...

From the moment I learned to walk, I was a hopelessly active child. If I wasn't out riding around the neighborhood on my bike or swimming in our backyard pool, I was doing gymnastics on the front lawn or (despite my father's protests) down the carpeted hallway that opened to our living room. There were diving contests, games of badminton, and baseball games using an old wooden bat my mom had used growing up in the 1930s. I rarely sat still, except to do homework and watch *Rin Tin Tin* every day at 4:30.

In the fourth grade, my parents enrolled me in competitive gymnastics so I would have a structured outlet for some of my energy. I competed for four years but realized once I went to high school that I didn't have time for two-hour practices four days a week plus the mounds of homework the Sisters of Mercy were giving us at school. About the same time, I also took a nasty fall on the balance beam. Although I wasn't seriously injured, that was the first time I ever came close to getting hurt and it introduced me to a previously unknown sense of fear. When asked by my parents if I wanted to continue competing, it didn't take much thought to decide I wanted to focus more on my studies and less on my future as a gymnast, which I saw as fleeting anyway.

About a year or so after I quit gymnastics, my best friend and I went by our former gym to say hello to the coaches. I can remember it like it was yesterday. I was standing in the viewing area, looking out over the gym behind the plexiglass window, watching the new generation of girls tumble and flip while we waited for the coaches to finish talking to some parents in the office. One of the coaches – the one with whom we all had a love-hate relationship because of his militant approach to coaching – finished his conversation first and came up behind us. The first words out of his mouth were in reference to the size of my butt and the fact that it was "too large to do gymnastics now anyway."

We all have moments in our lives that we will never forget. They may be memories of actual events etched so indelibly in our Minds that we can play them back in vivid detail, or they may be the recollection of words that were said to us. No matter their form, these moments have a profound impact on us and the course of our lives from that point forward.

This was one of those moments.

I was in the throes of puberty, battling hormones and the realization that my body wasn't metabolizing the foods I once ate in quite the same way that it used to, especially now that I wasn't training in the gym four days a week and wasn't quite as active as I had always been. I was already self-conscious on every level that a normal teenage girl is self-conscious and in less than 10 seconds, this grown man had added a whole other level of self-consciousness to the mix.

I don't remember anything else about that visit that day. I just know I never went back there.

It wasn't long after that – possibly that summer – when an equally insensitive uncle saw me at a family event. I was standing in the kitchen of his Lake Ontario cottage, a place where I had spent so many fun and relaxing summers running around on the rocks by the water, fishing, riding dirt bikes, and being the active kid I described above. With one loud exclamation, made in front of other aunts, uncles and cousins, he shattered those memories and replaced them with a more lasting one of him declaring, "Look at the dupa on her!"

I am 100% Polish, and for those who don't know, "dupa" is Polish for "butt."

So here we were again with comments being made about my butt.

Mind you, I wasn't obese. I was 5'2" and 115 pounds. Admittedly, I carried more of that weight in my derriere than elsewhere but it wasn't like my gymnastics coach and my uncle were showcasing rock-hard physiques and had any right to pass judgment on anyone, especially a girl going through the hormonal changes of a teenager.

I am sure they had no idea the impact of their words but those two incidents set the stage for what would become years upon years of calorie-counting and dieting. I can still remember packing a bag of yogurt-covered "fruit snacks" (thinking the 100-calorie bags were healthy) and a couple of rice cakes for lunch every day in high school. I'd eat breakfast but either skip or only nibble on dinner. Tumbling down the hallway was replaced by nightly ab exercises in that same hall, where the carpeting was easier on my back than were the hardwoods we had elsewhere in the house (this, by the way, made my father no happier than my tumbling because now he had to be careful not to step on me when rounding a blind corner from the kitchen!).

Not much about my diet was nutritious or healthy, but by the time I went off to college, I had dropped at least 10 pounds and no longer sported a big dupa…and frankly, at that stage in my life, that was all that mattered.

Unfortunately, however, my dieting obsession didn't stop there. Not only did my caloric restrictions continue after I went off to school but I also discovered the gym and began weight lifting and doing cardio on a daily basis. Before I graduated college, I had dropped below 90 pounds and was surviving on Diet Coke, a sleeve of saltine crackers (400 calories per sleeve, for anyone wondering), Double Bubble chewing gum, and 1-hour workouts per day, every day.

I wish I could say I was kidding but…I'm not.

It was only when I came home to visit my parents during my senior year and my dad sat beside me with tears in his eyes and asked me to stop whatever I was doing that it started to occur to me that I had gone too far. Shortly thereafter, an ex-boyfriend saw me on campus and echoed my dad's sentiments, telling me he didn't recognize me and that I was just too thin.

These moments were as pivotal as the ones involving my coach and my uncle and probably saved my life.

During my 20s, I worked on finding a healthy balance in my life, eating more nutritious foods in combination with reasonable amounts of exercise, so that I could add healthy pounds to my frame. I had a job that involved traveling every week so there were challenges involved in making healthy selections from restaurant menus but that was probably a blessing at the time. I was forced to eat more balanced meals than I might otherwise have done if left to my own devices. There were ups and downs in the process and my wardrobe included pants in four different sizes but I was at least heading in the right direction overall.

It really wasn't until I reached my 30s that things began to stabilize. However, even then, each day continued to be a battle with food and whenever I overindulged, I punished myself with longer workouts to make up for it.

Now, in my 40s, I have come to understand that

weight loss and weight management do not have to be a constant struggle and that loving and nurturing our bodies does a lot more good than punishing them. Though I have come within a couple years of personally proving true the statistic that the average woman spends 31 years of her life on a diet, I am finally free of the dieting mentality and living a healthy lifestyle that is actually fun and enjoyable. This book reflects the many lessons I had to learn to reach this point and includes many of the tools that I personally used and continue to use each day in my approach to healthy living.

And Now...A Little About You

If you're reading this book, I'm going to assume you're in the process of trying to lose weight or are thinking about climbing aboard the proverbial Weight Loss Wagon to embark on a weight-loss journey. And if you're like most people, this probably isn't your first trip. You've probably been on and off the Wagon multiple times and may have so many Frequent Rider points that you now qualify for Chairman's Preferred status! Your story and what led you to where you are today will not be the same as my story but I am willing to bet that something in my story resonated with you or that our stories share some similarities.

When it comes to weight loss, today's media floods us with information. For the most part, we know what to do (and what not to do) in terms of exercise and healthy eating (much more than I knew when I thought a bag of yogurt-covered fruit snacks was a healthy lunch option!). So why is it that so many of us still struggle year after year to win the weight-loss battle? What are we missing and what can we do about it?

To paraphrase something my mother used to tell me as a child, "If you understand the Mind, you'll understand everything."

The Mind is where it's at. It's what controls our emotions, our thoughts, our behaviors, our decisions, everything. It's also what keeps us on or off the Weight Loss Wagon. Although weight loss certainly depends on healthy eating and exercise, it's the Mind that controls our decisions to do those things…to make the right choices in the first place. It's the precursor to all the other stuff.

And what's the one thing missing from cookie-cutter diets and basic workout programs?

Yup. You guessed it. The mindset element.

The internet is loaded these days with weight-loss resources, many of which are free of charge, and we all know about brand-name weight-loss companies like Weight Watchers, Jenny Craig and Nutrisystem. To supplement nutritional guidance, the personal training industry has grown dramatically in recent years, so there is no shortage of qualified individuals to help us design and stick to a workout plan to complement our eating patterns.

This book isn't about any of those things. It's not about meal plans or food. It doesn't get into the great debate as to whether cardio or weight training is better for you. It's not going to inundate you with fat-loss statistics and science that blow your Mind with such force that any hope of implementing the underlying guidelines is lost in the puff of smoke that trails behind. This book assumes that you have already done your homework and found a healthy eating and exercise plan that works for you. You may have hired a nutrition professional and/or a personal trainer to help you, or you may have flown solo and designed your plans on your own. Regardless, the assumption is that you're ready to get started. All you need to do is pull the trigger and fire the starting shot.

Sooo...if this book isn't about the fundamentals of weight loss that countless other books

address, what IS this book about?

This book is about focus and sustainable motivation.

It's about getting and keeping your head in the game during the first 30 days of your weight-loss journey so you can make changes that stick.

And it's about support.

Strong support systems are essential for permanent weight loss but not all of us are blessed with family and friends who understand our weight-loss goals. In fact, our friends and family may even feel threatened by our aspirations. This book is written to make you go deep and find your inner cheerleader. That cheerleader will become your best friend.

YOU will become your best friend.

And once that happens, look out – the impossible becomes possible!

When you are truly able to connect with your innermost desires and work in harmony with them, that's when the magic starts to happen!

From my experience, the first 30 days of adjusting to a change are always the toughest, primarily because of the mental barriers that automatically go up whenever our Mind realizes that the status quo is about to shift. At some point during the 30 days, you're likely to feel the full spectrum of emotions known to humankind – everything from fear to excitement, anger to acceptance, sadness to happiness, frustration to satisfaction.

If you're from my generation, you may even, on occasion, hear the voice of Jim McKay echoing in your head, commenting about the "thrill of victory and the agony of defeat" as if your journey is the weight-loss equivalent of ABC's *Wide World of Sports* and you are the unfortunate skier tumbling down the mountain every time you have an ill-fated relapse (and relapses WILL happen, even to the best of us!).

When you think about it in emotional terms, it's really no wonder so many of us fall off the Weight Loss Wagon. Processing so many emotions in a relatively short span of time can be overwhelming for even the most detached and unaffecting individual, and once our emotions get the best of us, off the Wagon we go.

The Mind keeps us balanced and even-keeled.

In the following chapters you will find motivation and inspiration to take you from Day 1 through Day 30 of your weight-loss journey. Each chapter will offer tips and tricks for managing the emotions you're likely to experience and keep you from falling into common pitfalls.

Think of this book as your bedside companion...or as your personal coach...and know that each page is ready and waiting to offer words of encouragement and reassurance. All you have to do is make use of it!

Every day for the next 30 days, commit to reading at least one chapter. Perhaps you will want to wake up and read a chapter in the morning to jumpstart your day. Maybe you'll find more value in reading at night before bedtime, when you can reflect on the day's events. You can read the chapters in order or you can jump around and read whatever chapter resonates with you best on any given day. Although I tried to transition from one chapter to the next based on typical emotions experienced throughout the 30-day window, we all know: there's no such thing as "typical," especially when it comes to emotions! For this reason, each chapter is designed to be read on its own without requiring that you have read the chapter before it. The first and last chapters are the only ones I would recommend you read on the suggested days (Days 1 and 30). Beyond that, how you read and use this book is up to you!

To help you decide if a particular day's message is relevant for you, each chapter begins with a Mood Indicator. Just like a forecast predicts the weather, the Mood Indicator predicts the emotions you will likely face during the first 30 days of your journey. The content of each day's message digs deeper into those emotions and teaches you coping skills to prevent such feelings from stalling or stopping your weight-loss journey.

I've intentionally given you a lot of flexibility for using this book as a mindset resource to complement whatever eating and/or exercise plans you have chosen. All you have to do is commit to using it and then brace yourself to see how changes that you never before could make soon become healthy new habits you will love for life!

And now, without further ado, let's get this journey started!

DAY 1: You're On Your Way!

MOOD INDICATOR: Feeling mostly excited but also feeling fear and self-doubt

ALOHA!

No, I am not Hawaiian…and this book has nothing to do with Hawaii…but who doesn't feel a surge of positive emotions when they hear that beautiful Hawaiian greeting?

"Aloha" is one of those words that just makes us inexplicably happy (and the associated vision of being kicked back in a lounge chair, flaunting a hot new body, umbrella drink in hand, doesn't hurt either!).

Today is the first day of your weight-loss journey and although you're certain to be excited, you're also going to be faced with a whirlwind of emotions and second-guessing, wondering things like:

"Do I *really* want to do this?"

"Am I *really* ready to make changes?"

"What if I can't stick to my eating plan or I cave into temptation on a regular basis?"

"I have so much going on in my life – do I really want to tackle this now? Maybe I should just wait a while and see if I start to lose weight on my own, without following a formal program."

Whenever we start something new, it's natural to have reservations and some degree of self-doubt, but amidst the racket of voices clamoring in your head at the start of this journey, it's important to remember that you've already made what will probably be the hardest decision of the entire weight-loss process: you've made the initial decision to change your habits and to lose weight. No matter how big or small, change, by its very nature, is scary but you've confronted that dreaded four-letter "f" word (fear!) and committed to change anyway.

So take a deep breath, let out a sigh of relief that one of the hardest decisions is behind you, and start your journey with a happiness-infused "ALOHA!" to displace your doubts and second-guessing!

The literal meaning of "aloha" is "the presence of breath" or "the breath of life." In fact, many Hawaiians view aloha as a way of living and treating each other with respect, starting with a solid foundation of self-love that can then be spread to others. According to the old Hawaiian priests, living the spirit of aloha is a way of living in harmony with the Universe such that you become a source of positive energy.

Whether you know this yet or not, by embarking on a weight-loss journey and electing to use this book as your mindset resource, you're bound to reach new levels of self-realization. During the upcoming weeks, you are going to reclaim (or maybe discover for the first time) a relationship with your body and what it needs and wants. You will start to notice habits you may not have realized you had or food triggers you didn't know existed. You're going to find new ways to live in harmony with your body and establish a more nurturing relationship with it. You'll transform negative thought patterns into positive ones and you will likely find that amazing things start to happen as your greater self-awareness guides you in living a lifestyle that promotes sustainable weight loss.

Your journey is, in fact, going to lead you closer to living the spirit of aloha!

So kick self-doubt and anxiety to the curb, dear reader, and get excited!

You're about to go on a journey that will not only transform your body but also your approach to life…and it's gonna be awesome!

MINDSET TOOL:

If you haven't already done so, take out a sheet of paper and write down your weight-loss and weight-loss-related goals. Until you write down your goals, all you really have are intentions, but the simple act of writing something down has an odd way of fostering commitment and transforming those intentions into true goals.

You can handwrite your goals on a piece of paper or, if you're used to using Word or PowerPoint, you can document them electronically, perhaps using a snazzy font and background template. The more you can turn this small exercise into a mini project and add personal touches, the more you will promote true ownership of your goals and their achievement.

Next, post your goals somewhere you will see them every day for the next 30 days. That may be on your refrigerator, on your bathroom mirror or vanity counter, or at the front of your daily planner. If you don't mind sharing with the world, you may even make them your screen saver! These written goals will serve as visual reminders of why you started your journey and what you want to accomplish by the end, and visual reminders can be tremendously powerful. If you don't believe me, think about the reason people decorate weeks in advance for Halloween, Christmas and other holidays. Holiday decorations create visual reminders that festive times are coming, and these reminders, in turn, influence the subconscious and usually boost everyone's spirits. In like manner, seeing your written goals on a regular basis will subconsciously influence you and help keep you on the Weight Loss Wagon.

In the event that self-doubt and fear sneak into your consciousness despite your best efforts to discourage them, remind yourself that today and every day (for the next 30 days as well as every day for the rest of your life), you have the power of choice.

Just as you started this journey by choice, you can, at any time along the way, stop or hit "pause."

You always have free will, and this is YOUR journey. Own it and make it the best journey possible but at the same time, don't forget that you are in the driver's seat and have control. Sometimes simply remembering that will be all it takes to keep fear at bay, keep you motivated and keep you on track.

By embarking on this journey, huge possibilities and immensely positive things are now at your fingertips. Give yourself a mental high five for taking the initiative to claim them as your own then set your focus, get your Mind in the game, and get started!

DAY 2: Culinary Panic Attacks
MOOD INDICATOR: Feeling straight-up panic!

It doesn't matter if it's Day 2 or Day 25. There are going to be days when you have what I call Culinary Panic Attacks. These insidious attacks usually hit you out of nowhere. You may be coasting along just fine, thinking how it hasn't been all that bad adjusting to new eating habits and workout routines. Then suddenly, somewhere in the shadows of your Mind, you hear it. A little voice pecking away at your Left Brain, trying to gain entry by pretending it's the Voice of Reason (I told you it was insidious!). It doesn't even use big, impressive words. It just talks trash like "Is this how it's gonna be for the rest of my life? Am I *NEVER* going to be able to eat another [*insert your favorite less-than-healthy food here*]???!"

And that's all it takes.

Anxiety turns into panic.

Panic turns into despair.

And the next thing you know you're grabbing for the bag of *Chips Ahoy!,* rationalizing that life was meant to be enjoyed and by God, you're gonna enjoy it!

Well, at least in the heat of the feeding frenzy.

Post-frenzy…probably within just minutes of eating the last cookie…you'll likely find yourself morphing from the champion of "carpe diem" ("live for the day") into the poster child for "amitte diem," or "let the opportunity pass."

Why, oh why, couldn't you have just let the opportunity to devour all those cookies pass?!!!

Culinary Panic Attacks are sneaky but they are not invincible.

When you feel one coming on, first recognize it for what it is. Culinary Panic Attacks are not founded in logic or reality. They are merely your imagination running wild and getting the best of you.

That said, you may indeed discover that avoiding certain foods is your secret to maintaining permanent weight loss. Everyone has trigger foods that either make them gain weight or make them eat more (which, obviously, makes them gain weight). Avoiding these foods certainly helps to keep weight off once you've lost it. However, if you are following an appropriate and healthy diet/meal plan to lose the weight in the first place, no food should be banned for life (unless you have an allergy or some other medical condition, of course). To this point...

It will always be <u>your choice</u> as to whether you eat the food or pass it up. No one can take that choice from you, so you can see that panicking over *never again* being "allowed" to eat something doesn't make a lot of sense.

Furthermore, if you are following a healthy weight-loss plan that's tailored for your body and lifestyle, the plan will likely include periods of greater dietary restriction in the beginning, followed by periods of greater freedom that ultimately lead to a more liberal maintenance plan. When you think of weight loss in terms of this process – adhering to the most restrictive period first, followed by a less restrictive period, followed by long-term maintenance with the least amount of restriction – you can more readily squelch panicky emotions because you know that your journey has boundaries and that you have control at all times.

Once you lose the weight you set out to lose, you should be able to transition to a healthy, sustainable eating plan that will allow occasional indulgences. (Note: If your plan is not designed this way, you may want to consider another plan.)

Foods in and of themselves are not inherently good or bad. Some have more nutritional value than others. Some have more caloric value than others. However, it's the choices we make about the quantities we consume, when we consume, and the other foods/beverages with which we consume any given food, in combination with our own genetic and metabolic profile, that determine the impact of the food on our weight. If there is a food you think you simply cannot live without, don't panic. You can try adding it back into your meal plan in controlled quantities when the time in your journey is right. For now, when these Culinary Panic Attacks occur, simply remind yourself of this possibility, reclaim your choice to continue following your current plan, and keep an open Mind about possibly replacing the "I-can't-live-without" food with something healthier.

Think of your journey as a time to experiment with healthy stuff. Have fun and see what piques the interest of your taste buds.

You may be surprised to find that by the end of your journey, you no longer like the very foods that initially caused you to have Culinary Panic Attacks. (This actually happened to me when I abstained from wine during a 12-week weight-loss journey, prior to which I was seriously in love with wine; the very day I was allowed to have wine again, the taste repulsed me!).

MINDSET TOOL:

Aside from mentally going toe-to-toe with them when they occur and talking yourself off the ledge of irrational thinking, another tool for managing your Culinary Panic Attacks is to build a reward system into your weight-loss program. That said, realize upfront that there are differing opinions about the value of using food as a reward when you are trying to lose weight. Some find this to be risky business because it requires discipline and control in regard to something (food) that may have historically been difficult for you to control. Other schools of thought simply think we should be able to automatically turn off our taste buds and cravings so that we only want the things on our meal plan from this day forward, til death do us part. In fact, a trainer/nutrition consultant from this school of thought once chastised me for "being a puppy" when I wanted to include a single glass of my old friend, vino, as a culinary treat/reward in my program.

The puppy comparison was the last straw in a series of demeaning comments and I quit working with him later that month, as soon as my agreement expired. However, on the point of using culinary motivation in a structured weight-loss program, I also fundamentally disagreed with him.

For me – and I believe for most of us – there has to be something to which to look forward on the food horizon in order to incent us to remain "compliant" with the new eating habits we're adopting. Otherwise, it's more likely that we WILL succumb to a Culinary Panic Attack and spiral into an abyss of fear and overwhelming panic, causing us to make not just poor but outright TERRIBLE food choices. And who wins then? No one, except maybe the makers of that empty bag of *Chips Ahoy!* that you'll be tempted to replace for the next panic attack.

The knowledge that we will one day be able to have some of our former comfort foods, even in small quantities, has amazing motivational power.

If you are working with a nutrition professional who understands the reward system, you may already have "cheat meals" included throughout your plan. If not, talk to the person who created your meal plan and see if he/she is willing to incorporate some preemptive "cheats." If you are flying solo and using a diet or meal plan you found online or in a book, you may need to build your own cheat meals into the program.

Typically, cheat meals will occur once a week and they MUST be restricted to a single meal only. They are a cheat MEAL, not a cheat DAY. Furthermore, by my definition, cheat meals do not give you carte blanche to eat whatever the heck you want and can shovel in your mouth all in one sitting. They should be carefully designed to appease cravings by using controlled quantities of just one or two food items. For example, because I have (since the end of the 12-week program I mentioned above) reignited my love affair with wine, and because I consciously choose not to give it up for good, I allow myself one or two glasses every Friday night with dinner. Everything else about my eating patterns on Friday remains the same as any other day of the week. If anything, I compensate for my vino indulgence by being even more aware of what I eat throughout the day to ensure that my overall caloric intake stays tight. However, by allowing myself some Friday night wine, I give myself something to which to look forward and that makes it easier to stay compliant with my program every other day of the week.

Everyone is wired differently so cheats may or may not work for you but they are certainly a tool worth considering, particularly if you find yourself battling frequent Culinary Panic Attacks.

DAY 3: The Value of Timeouts

MOOD INDICATOR: Feeling stable and clear

Not every day of your weight-loss journey will be an emotional battlefield. There will be plenty of days when you feel content with your progress, your healthy new habits, and your overall program. But even on what I call the "stable and clear" days, it's important to remain vigilant about keeping your Mind actively involved in the weight-loss process.

One thing you can do on a "stable and clear" day is set up a framework for taking timeouts that will remind you to celebrate personal victories throughout your weight-loss journey.

Celebrating small things throughout your journey is crucial for long-term success, even if your first celebration occurs on your third day and all you're celebrating is the fact that you made it through Days 1 and 2. Every victory, however small, is HUGE in terms of keeping you on track and mentally engaged in your weight-loss program. If you're going it alone and have a limited support system, the need to acknowledge your accomplishments becomes even more important because no one is likely going to do that for you.

You can think of these celebrations as mental timeouts that allow you to momentarily stop *doing* your program so that you can review your progress to-date and give yourself a pat on the back. These are also opportunities to ensure that your strategy and actions continue to align.

Consider team sports. It's easy for players to get caught up in playing the game. Emotions run high and adrenaline is flowing. Attention is on the next move and scoring points. Yet, in just about every sports game out there, teams use timeouts to stop the clock. These timeouts give players a momentary rest on the physical plane but they do not disable or disrupt mental focus. To the contrary, they are usually called to give the team a pep talk and then help the team regroup and regain focus so that the next leg of the game can be played more efficiently and effectively.

When you're trying to change eating behaviors or adopt new workout routines, it's easy to place your attention on tactical things like preparing meals that fit your plan, measuring portions, drinking your daily allotment of water, etc. But you need to incorporate timeouts into the program as well. During these timeouts, you can celebrate your small victories by acknowledging the hard work and progress you've made. This acknowledgement can be as simple as reviewing your actions from the past few days and noting how many times you declined food items you were offered that were not on your meal plan. Or you can count the number of meals you ate that followed your plan's guidelines to a tee. Or maybe you recognize during your timeout that you went an entire day without taking any licks, bites or tastes of others' meals (for example, your kids' leftovers)...and you didn't even miss those extra calories one bit!

You can either write your accomplishments down in a journal or take a mental inventory and review them – whichever approach works best for you.

A celebration doesn't have to be over the top, particularly when it is a mental celebration. The Mind is easily encouraged; it's just that we often neglect its need for encouragement. Taking the time to think, "You know, I did a really good job yesterday!" goes a long way in terms of maintaining our long-term focus and helping us stay the course on our journey.

As an added bonus, taking timeouts and celebrating our mini-victories builds healthy self-esteem, which is critical to long-term weight management.

MINDSET TOOL:

You probably read this chapter and thought, "OK. Easy peasy. Remember to celebrate my victories, however small."

But before you move on to another chapter, I strongly recommend that you schedule time at least once a week for the next 30 days to take a timeout and reflect on your accomplishments. While it's easy to think right now that you will remember to do that without committing to it on a calendar, you will be amazed at how quickly the "easy stuff" will be forgotten or skipped as you try to maintain the hectic pace of life and also focus on your weight-loss journey.

Although you certainly can't predict when you might want to celebrate an unexpected accomplishment during the next 30 days (those will be "impromptu celebrations"), holding time on your calendar to pause and reflect will force you to recognize on a regular basis the small accomplishments that you may otherwise overlook or dismiss as insignificant. You can still celebrate the unpredictable accomplishments as they happen but taking planned timeouts helps turn the act of routinely reflecting / acknowledging / celebrating into a healthy mental habit.

Technology has made many of us slaves to our iPhones and email so use these devices to your advantage. It's easy to reserve 15 minutes each week on your calendar and set your alarm as a reminder to take your timeouts. If you're more traditional, you can ink the 15-minute blocks in your personal planner. Once the activity is planned, it becomes less likely that you will skip or forget it and soon you'll find it's become a valuable part of your weekly routine.

DAY 4: What Superhero Are You?

MOOD INDICATOR: Feeling alone and a little weak

At some point in your life, you've probably heard someone ask the question, "If you could be any superhero you wanted to be, which one would you be and why?"

This exercise is often used as an "ice breaker" for corporate team-building functions. The intent of the exercise is typically to better understand the personality traits of individual team members based on how they relate to those of well-known superheroes. By sharing the results of either formal "superhero quizzes" or individual self-assessments with an entire team, members of the team are better able to understand each other's strengths and weaknesses and leverage individual strengths for the benefit of the entire group.

There will be days on your weight-loss journey when you're going to wish you had the benefit of being part of a larger team…when you wish you were just a single cog in a wheel and that how far you progress and where you end up didn't depend solely on you. Sure, you may be receiving help from the professionals who designed your program, but you boarded the Weight Loss Wagon alone. Your trainer can't and isn't going to do the workouts for you and your nutritionist can't make your meals and put the food in your mouth.

You're it, baby! You're a team of one!

Here's the good news.

You know those voices in your head? (It's OK – you can admit to having them. We all do and it doesn't make us crazy!) You can put those voices to work for you.

At least one of them represents a personality that says, "I can do this! I can do ANYTHING I set my Mind to!" Now, it may be a long time since you've heard this voice because it may have been muffled by the others that have been mumbling cynical thoughts about hopelessness, despair and the drudgery of life. But I promise you. That voice is in you. It's there. Your job is to pull it up to the surface and let it talk.

One way to help yourself do this is to consider which superhero this voice most resembles…or that you WANT it to resemble (hey, it's YOUR inner voice…make it what you want!).

MINDSET TOOL:

I have listed below some of the most popular superheroes and their powers. Use this list or any list you want (you can search online) to find the superhero to whom you can most relate and whose super powers you think would help you. This superhero should also be the one you want to associate with your inner voice of encouragement throughout your weight-loss journey.

Find a picture of this superhero and print it out. Carry that picture with you or put it in a place where you will frequently see it. Use the picture as a visual reminder that, although your biggest fan, your biggest cheerleader, and your biggest source of power is YOU, you also have a superhero within you that will help you every step of the way in realizing your full potential. Use him/her as your secret weapon in times of need.

It may even help to talk to your superhero. Let's say you decide your inner superhero is Wonder Woman.

One of Wonder Woman's super powers was her immunity to illusions and Mind control. So the next time you're feeling tempted to binge on a pint of ice cream or indulge in a plate full of French fries, why not try talking to your inner Wonder Woman? It doesn't have to be an elaborate conversation. All the conversation may need to involve is the thought that Wonder Woman would be able to resist the Mind tricks being played on you by the ice cream or French fries, so "C'mon, Inner Wonder Woman! Help me resist as well!"

Calling on your inner superhero and reminding yourself of your inner strength may very well give you the push you need to get past the hurdle of temptation unscathed.

Associating behaviors with mental images can be quite powerful. Just thinking about resisting temptation is one thing but when you think about doing that AND have a mental image to go along with it – something like the image of Wonder Woman using her powers to push away temptations – you suddenly give yourself a mental edge.

If you have a particular aversion to superheroes, think of some other figure you admire and who will inspire you to stay the course during your weight-loss journey.

Perhaps you adore Carrie Bradshaw from the famous *Sex and the City* series and wish you had half her confidence and charisma. Use her character as your inspiration, just as you would a superhero. It's all about what works for you!

This tool also reminds you that all the tools and resources you need really DO exist within you. Don't be afraid to tap into them and draw them out. Kids do this all the time. Their imaginations are usually very active and enhance their lives greatly. Unfortunately, adults are conditioned to suppress these abilities, but it's time to end the suppression. **Put the power of imagination to work for you!**

Super Power	Superhero
Ability to heal rapidly	Wolverine
Invisibility	Invisible Woman
Superhuman endurance	Tick
Superhuman agility	Blade
Superhuman senses	Supergirl
Superhuman strength	Hulk
Vision-based power	Superman
Superhuman speed	Flash
Elasticity	Plastic Man

DAY 5: Let's Have a Party! (A Pity Party, That Is....)

MOOD INDICATOR: Feeling sorry for yourself

The real world is not like *Extreme Makeover: Weight Loss* or *The Biggest Loser*. If you're like most people, "regularly scheduled programming" (i.e., your day-to-day responsibilities and life) will not be interrupted for you to go off and focus solely on your weight-loss journey. You are going to have to make the journey while simultaneously juggling your family duties, work responsibilities, household chores, and a myriad of other things for which you will remain accountable despite embarking on this trip.

You can't put life on hold.

And sometimes…this won't seem fair.

You'll start to look around and wonder why you have

to do this…why are you the one prone to weight gain when you so much as LOOK at a cookie, but your sister can eat an entire bag of cookies and not gain an ounce? Why did your metabolism have to change from your 20s to your 40s when you see middle-aged models and actresses sprawled across the pages of magazines, seemingly immune to the impacts of the aging process? How did you get dealt this crappy hand of cards?

Pity parties are fairly common during a weight-loss journey. You're inevitably going to have times when you just want to say "uncle" and demand to know why it is that you can't be naturally thin and carefree.

Let me stop you right there.

First off, "thin" doesn't necessarily mean "carefree." Whether you are 20 pounds overweight or 20 pounds underweight or exactly at your ideal weight, happiness will only follow if you've reached a place of contentment within yourself.

Many of the exercises included in this book are intended to teach you to appreciate the gifts you have within…not the number you reach on the scale or the size clothing you wear.

The outer package doesn't define you and it certainly doesn't guarantee any degree of happiness. We all know beautiful people who appear to be walking perfection to the outside world but live in states of extreme unhappiness in the privacy of their homes.

So now that we have cleared up that "thin" and "carefree" are not synonymous, I want you to also banish the idea of someone being "naturally thin." We were all given different body types. Each one is unique and defines what we are "naturally" supposed to be. Yes, some body types are thinner than others and probably always will be, but when you start talking about "naturally thin" vs. "naturally heavy," the implication is that one person was given a superior set of genes over the other...and that's completely untrue!

We all have awesome genes with features, talents and abilities unique unto us...and that's pretty damn cool!

So rather than dwell on the body type that you have versus the one that your sister or cousin or best friend or the magazine model has...and rather than put that person's body type on a pedestal...why not instead focus on the fact that you were given a body with tons of potential, just like everyone else? It's now up to you to manifest that potential by giving your body the love and attention it needs to be its healthiest.

And if you're still looking for a reason to throw the pity party you were hell-bent on throwing at the start of this chapter, I'm now going to close with a healthy dose of tough love:

As far as your weight-loss journey is concerned, you're not a victim…and no amount of pity partying and no argument you make will ever convince me otherwise.

You were given kick-ass genes and amazing potential but your choices in the past have resulted in less than optimal results. It's now time to face the music and take charge of the situation you created, not wallow in moments of unfounded self-pity.

Ouch.

I know it stings, but someone has to tell you the truth even when it's hard to bear.

MINDSET TOOL:

Although they will happen, there is really no time for pity parties on the road to weight loss and wellness. If you find yourself slipping into one, you have to break that party up before it gets out of hand. You have your challenges (one of which is weight) but everyone else has challenges, too. Don't allow yourself to wallow in an unjustified sense of sorrow.

As a mental exercise to help you combat moments of self-pity, I want you to think about the reasons you're on this weight-loss journey. What really put you here? Your genetics may have played a role in your bone structure and frame but when you cut through the bullshit (pardon my language but that's exactly what this is), your choices played the greatest role in putting extra weight on your body. Your choices to eat processed foods instead of whole foods, to eat too much of all foods, to avoid the gym like the plague, to live off soda and Skittles, to make fun of your sister when she asked if you wanted to take yoga with her. Choices like that are what led you to where you are today.

Take ownership of those choices and stop playing the victim.

I'm not in any way saying you should chastise yourself or beat yourself up. All I am saying is that you need to own the responsibility once and for all, then commit to making things right from here on out.

When you feel the urge to feel sorry for yourself, remind yourself that your choices and your decisions are what led you to where you are today but they are also what will lead you to where you want to be tomorrow.

This moment, and every moment forward, offers a fresh start. What you do with the moment and the opportunity is entirely up to you.

DAY 6: Permission to Fail

MOOD INDICATOR: Feeling discouraged, aggravated and frustrated with yourself

One of the best gifts you can give yourself during your weight-loss journey is the permission to fall short or plain old screw up.

Before you start yelling, "Wait? What? What kind of a beside companion and coach are you? You're supposed to be boosting my confidence, telling me I'm gonna make it…not telling me it's OK to screw up!"…please. Just hear me out.

For anyone trying something new – whether it's a more structured fitness routine or a new way of eating or simply a new way of looking at food – the ability to allow oneself to mess up and, dare I say, to even *expect* to mess up, is invaluable to long-term success.

As humans, we are not perfect. Intellectually, we know

this. After all, there is a reason for the age-old saying, "Practice makes perfect." Yet, how many of us set different expectations for ourselves when we try something new? For whatever reason, we think we need to pole vault past any kind of learning curve and achieve instant gratification and success. And very often, if we don't succeed right out of the gate, we throw away the entire idea as foolish or just not meant to be.

Crazy, huh?

But quite often true!

As you begin to adopt changes in your eating and exercise behavior, you will inevitably have "good" days and "bad" days. There will be days when you stay the course and stick with your action plan 100%, but there may be other days when, for whatever reason, you get distracted or fall a little short of your self-imposed targets. At those times, it is crucial that you allow yourself permission to do that.

To be human.

To screw up.

People in the process of change often "throw the baby out with the bath water" as soon as they hit a bump in the road. One small slip-up (or two or three) sends them spiraling downward, blaming themselves for being a failure and deciding there is no point in continuing to try.

Nothing could be further from the truth!

Behavioral change (including changes in eating and workout behavior) is no different than learning to ride a bike. You aren't going to hop on and ride 10 miles on your first day. More likely, you are going to hop on, fall off, scrape your knee, fall a few more times, scrape an elbow, and maybe ride up and down the driveway before calling it a day. But you will practice some more on the second day, and the third day, and so on…and eventually you WILL hop on and be able to ride 10 miles if that's what you want to do.

When we have realistic expectations set and accept that making mistakes and falling short is all just part of the long-term process, our odds for success improve exponentially. As you embrace new habits, remember to be gentle with yourself and view each mis-step as merely a stepping stone and each day as another day of practice. This isn't about perfection so there's really no need to put that extra pressure on yourself. This is about becoming the best YOU that you can be!

MINDSET TOOL:

The entire weight-loss journey, including its slips and falls, is about YOU, so there is no blueprint for doing it "right." The following checklist highlights the important mindset elements that underlie most successful journeys. In the event that you have a slip or fall, use this list to help you get back on track and refocus your energy.

Accept where you are today without judgment or shame or any other negative emotion.

You likely took this step before deciding to start your journey. If you did not, or if feelings of judgment or shame have surfaced after a slip or fall in your program, take a moment now to accept yourself. Close your eyes and think about the state of your body and health right now, pushing any negative feelings that may surface up and outside of yourself. Visualize those thoughts and feelings as being in front of you then encircle them in your Mind's eye with a bubble. You can color the bubble if you'd like but the intent is to encase the negative thoughts in a contained space then send them loving, healing energy and affirm in your

Mind that you will heal these thoughts by continuing the journey you've begun. Whenever you find yourself thinking negatively about yourself, do this quick exercise to detach from those thoughts, put them outside of yourself and regain control. It's shocking how much lighter you feel once the burden of those thoughts is taken from within and moved outside of you. The power of visualization should not be underestimated!

Establish written goals.

If you have not formally set your goals and written them down, refer to the Mindset Tool explained for Day 1 and do so now. If you have already done this exercise, re-read and recommit to your documented goals.

You've got tools – use 'em!

Your meal and/or exercise plans as well as this book and all of the tools suggested within each chapter constitute your toolkit. Think of them as life preservers that will come to your rescue whenever you slip or fall, and don't be afraid to use them. Try as many of the mindset tools you can and continually seek ways to build your toolkit by experimenting on your own.

Give yourself permission to make mistakes along the way.

No explanation required. Just do it and do it with conviction. Leave the guilt, shame and negative emotions at the door and replace them with a sense of curiosity. Make every mistake an opportunity to learn something about yourself and use that knowledge to prevent yourself from making the same mistakes in the future.

Practice, practice, practice your new habits, reminding yourself, when necessary, that it's OK not be perfect!

In fact, it's often in our imperfections that we discover secrets to help us stick with our plans longer and achieve greater results than we ever thought possible.

There will be trial and error, success and failure, and everything in between, but through practice and persistence, you'll be moving in the right direction for achieving sustainable success.

DAY 7: Can I Get a Little Persistence?

MOOD INDICATOR: Feeling challenged

Persistence is defined by Oxford Dictionaries as "firm or obstinate continuance in a course of action in spite of difficulty or opposition."

Virtually everyone following a weight-loss program is going to face unexpected obstacles and opposition somewhere along the way.

That's just life.

And life sometimes likes to throw a few extra curve balls into the mix to test your mettle. Maybe you have sustained an injury that prevents you from following your workout plan. Maybe your boss has loaded you up with so much work that finding time to prepare your meals and hit the gym seems virtually impossible.

In order to prevail in the face of unexpected

circumstances, you have to tap into your inner strength and persistence and resist self-sabotaging thoughts. You may hear yourself think such things as "I'll never lose weight, especially now that I am injured!" Or "This is stupid. I can't juggle my career and lose weight at the same time. Why did I think I could?"

If you continue to give these thoughts a voice in your head, however small, you will eventually believe them. During the first 30 days of your weight-loss journey, it is important to be particularly vigilant in your guard against negative thought patterns. When such notions begin to surface, try replacing them with constructive ways of thinking, such as, "My job may be more demanding right now and I may need to adjust my workout schedule a bit, but it's only temporary and not a reason to give up altogether." Or "I can't increase my physical activity right now because of my injury but I can continue to improve my eating habits and work on things that I CAN control."

You have to stick to the task until it's done.

To lose weight – whether it's five pounds or 55 pounds – you must exhibit persistence. You must accept that weight loss will take time (after all, you didn't gain the weight overnight and therefore should not expect to lose it overnight), and you must be willing to do the work required, even in the face of obstacles. Sometimes doing the work required may mean that you have to be creative (for example, working "around" an injury by doing different activities than you originally planned or adjusting your workout schedule to temporarily accommodate longer hours at the office), but the important thing is to continue doing it and not give up.

MINDSET TOOL:

The Mind can be trained to be persistent.

If you're facing some unexpected challenges on your weight-loss journey, take out a sheet of paper right now and make a chart with two columns: one for Walls (Obstacles) and one for Doors (New Opportunities).

In the first column, I want you to list everything you currently consider to be a wall or an obstacle to losing weight or sticking with your wellness plans. In the second column, I want you to explain how you will change that wall into a doorway to new opportunities.

For example:

Walls (Obstacles)	Doors (New Opportunities)
Example #1: Foot injury	• The foot injury limits the amount of walking I can do but I can do the recumbent bike instead. • Because I won't be able to do as much physical activity, this injury will also give me more time to focus on my eating habits and make healthy meals in advance.
Example #2: My kids' athletic practices and games will cut into my workout schedule	• Being unable to workout as much simply means that my eating habits have to be tighter and better than ever before. • Having to take the kids to sporting events in the evening just means I need to do my workouts first thing in the morning.

You've heard me say it already but the power of writing things down can be tremendous. This isn't a hard exercise to do. Give up 10 minutes of your time to brainstorm ideas then get to work on renovating your walls into doors!

DAY 8: Complacency

MOOD INDICATOR: Feeling comfortable and maybe even a little smug

One of the greatest threats to sustainable weight loss can sometimes be your progress and success.

Consider this scenario: You're cruising along, following your eating and exercise plans and beginning to see the pounds drop. Your clothes feel a little less snug. Your face looks a little leaner and less bloated. You know you haven't reached your goals yet but you're making progress and that's more than you've done in a long time. You feel on top of the world!

Initially, these kinds of feelings fuel your motivation and make you want to do even better…to adhere to your plans even more closely…to maybe do some extra walking or other exercise…to measure every serving of food right down to the nearest gram…or do other things to further your progress. I mean, whatever you're doing has obviously been working so why not try even harder? And so you do, and the results follow.

But somewhere along the way, you're not even sure when, those same feelings of exhilaration about your success suddenly stopped motivating you and made you become complacent. Whereas you were thinking just the other day how you couldn't live without your digital scale to keep your portions in check, you suddenly find yourself snubbing the very tool you had been praising as indispensable, thinking, "I really don't need to be THAT anal. I can eyeball it and be all right now." Or else you discover that you're sneaking in extra spoonfuls from the serving dish or having a glass of wine every night with dinner, rationalizing that these little things won't hurt. After all, you're ahead of your own expectations. You've been doing fabulous so a little cheating here and there won't do any harm.

And it may not do harm at first, but over the course of time (which may be just a few days), loosening the reigns in an uncontrolled manner (i.e., when not done as part of a structured program's transition to maintenance eating) WILL backfire on you, leaving you bewildered and frantic when you do your next weigh-in and realize you've gained back more than just a pound or two of "water weight."

There's a reason why the ancients had a proverb warning that the complacency of fools will destroy them!

MINDSET TOOL:

If you've lost some weight but find yourself starting to cut corners on your plan (shortening workouts or skipping them altogether, eyeballing portions, taking extra licks or bites after eating your meal, etc.), STOP and recommit. It's as simple as that. Pull out your written goals document from Day 1 and read it again. Read it WORD FOR WORD. Remind yourself of the reasons you committed to your weight-loss program and the fact that you have not yet reached the goals you set out to achieve. Yes, you've done well but there is still work to do and now is not the time to scale it down. Now is the time to turn it up and see what you've really got in you!

We're not talking about the rest of your life here. We're not saying you need to be dialed in to the highest frequency for eternity. We're only talking about the immediate future…the next few weeks or months or however long your program was designed to be to reach your goals. We're talking about a finite period.

Eventually you will transition back to "normal" living when you will have more flexibility and less rigor, but for right now, structure is necessary for continued progress. You can't cheat the system, no matter how hard you try.

Now, let's say that you have re-read your goals document from Day 1 and you find yourself thinking, "Well, you know…I originally wanted to lose 25 pounds but now that I have lost 10, I feel pretty good…and maybe 25 was unrealistic anyway. I am happy having lost 10 and I just want to be 'normal' NOW!"

Two things may be going on:

*Possibility #1: To use one of my dad's favorite expressions, "You're full of condensed milk!" (This was his polite version of the more vulgar expression… "You're full of sh*t!")*

If you're thinking you're OK with your current weight loss and don't need to go any further, I want you to put yourself to the acid test of honesty. I want you to go in a room, close the door (the bathroom works great for this if you have an intrusive family!), and have a come-to-Jesus meeting with yourself. There is not a soul in the world who will ever know about this but you. Look yourself in the mirror if you have one handy and ask yourself if you're ready to call it quits on losing more weight because you're really and truly happy where you are, OR if it's because you're settling. And if you even feel the smallest sensation that you may be settling (you will know this sensation when you feel it...it makes you kind of cringe either in the lower left side of your chest, right below your heart, or in your stomach), force yourself to explain why you're settling. Are you afraid of making more progress? Or are you afraid you won't be able to make more progress – i.e., has your success to date set the bar so high for future success that it scares you? Or are you just plain tired and don't have it in you to continue right now?

Upon doing this kind of introspection, I am willing to bet that you will either build yourself back up and decide to continue your program or that you will put your program on temporary hold but that you won't quit altogether.

If, however, after performing this honest introspection, you find that you have legitimate reasons for wanting to put your program on hiatus or end your program early then...

Possibility #2: Maybe your goals really WERE unrealistic or too aggressive.

I won't discount that as being possible, but if you believe that, I encourage you to talk to the professional who designed your plan and get a second opinion. If he/she agrees, then ask for a revision to your eating plan that will allow you to transition into the maintenance phase of your program using controlled behaviors. Even if you find you're ready for the maintenance phase sooner than you first expected, I do not recommend that you do this transition based on your cravings and your personal desire to just loosen up parts of your program because you don't like those parts. Get help from a qualified resource to make the changes you need to make.

If you're working on your own, you should still have a maintenance phase included in your overall program. If you don't, start researching immediately and use the free resources available online to help put together a solid plan for transitioning to maintenance eating.

DAY 9: Patience Is a Virtue…Just Not One of Mine

MOOD INDICATOR: Feeling impatient

Anyone who knows me is well aware that I am not an inherently patient person. Patience is just one of the virtues I never felt particularly compelled to espouse! From a very young age, I was conditioned to aspire and to achieve…and, once I achieved, to then set the bar even higher for my next round of goals.

Onward, march! Always moving forward, never moving backward, and certainly not standing still.

That mantra worked well in carrying me through childhood into my teenage years and even into early adulthood. After all, there was so much to learn and do, and each round of accomplishments laid the foundation for more learning and more opportunities for achievement as I expanded my horizons.

Unfortunately, it is this same model of constant forward movement and an underlying desire for instant gratification that has often derailed many weight-loss and wellness-improvement plans.

How can that be, you ask? Shouldn't we approach our state of wellness with the same zest and passion we had as children aspiring to ditch the training wheels and take our first training-wheel-free bike ride?

The answer is – yes and no.

While passion and enthusiasm are undeniably valuable, if not critical, to the success of a weight-loss program, you need to bear in mind that, unlike many of the things you learned as a child or young adult, weight loss is not a linear exercise. There is no 1-2-3 process map to follow like there was when your mom or dad first taught you to ride a tricycle, then moved you to the bicycle with training wheels, then removed the training wheels altogether. **When it comes to attaining your optimal weight, there are infinite ways in which countless factors can interact and influence the number on the scale as well as your overall state of well-being.** Furthermore, unlike the child learning to ride a bike, you may, in some cases, have many years of bad habits that will require rewiring before real progress can be seen. As a result, it is important that you approach your weight-loss program with a large degree of patience: patience with your body to respond to the changes you are making, patience with your Mind to fully embrace and adopt the changes, and patience with the process and methodology itself...and that last thing may be the hardest of all to master.

If you're following the guidance of a nutrition professional or using information from another source, chances are that some of the guidelines in your meal or exercise plan may at times seem too basic or too simple to matter, particularly if you're not seeing progress as quickly as you'd like. You may find yourself doubting the methodology and the process and bending rules you think don't matter anyway.

Take water, for instance. Water is considered by most programs to be essential for weight loss, and many diet coaches suggest drinking upwards of 100 ounces per day when following a fat-loss program. In the beginning of your program, this may be a challenge but you step up to the plate. As the days pass though, you may find yourself growing weary of this hydration requirement, thinking, "This can't be all that important. I've been drinking my daily water requirement and the pounds aren't dropping off at record speeds, so will drinking one less bottle of water really matter?" Next thing you know, you find yourself bending the rules of your plan and sliding off the Weight Loss Wagon.

Here's a newsflash: Despite what diet and supplement companies may want you to believe, weight loss does NOT have to be complicated. There is no mysterious voodoo magic involved. For most of us, there are a handful of dietary guidelines that, when followed consistently, can result in dramatic changes. We just have to be patient and trust the process long enough for those dramatic results to manifest.

You've got to give your new behaviors and associated eating patterns a chance to displace the effects that years of bad habits may have had.

Patience is inherently required whenever a weight-loss initiative is started. Although excitement and enthusiasm for improving one's wellness are invaluable to your overall success and should not be squelched in any way, it's equally important to temper your zest and passion with a healthy dose of patience…to remember that the weight-loss process isn't always straightforward and linear…and to recall my dad's version of a well-known quote he used to love saying to me: "Rome really wasn't built in one day, honey…Rome really wasn't built in one day!"

MINDSET TOOL:

In order to foster patience and maintain your interest in following your weight-loss program, I want you to think about your program not only as a journey but as an experiment. In an ideal world, every tool and technique you use in your meal and exercise plan will work like a champ, but more realistically, you may find that your weight-loss journey turns into a process of trial and error and that some of the things you try in the first few days or weeks will not resonate with you and your body type. That's why meal plans and workout routines often need to be tweaked from one week to the next.

Because of the experimental, non-linear nature of the weight-loss process, it's easy to become impatient when you're not seeing the results you want, but indulging in emotions like impatience will – like emotions always do – bump you off the Weight Loss Wagon for good unless you find ways to master them.

One very good tool for managing impatience is to track your reactions to elements of your weight-loss program. You can do this in regard to meals, to workouts, or both. Tracking these reactions doesn't have to be done using any particular format. You can simply buy a small, spiral-bound notebook that you can carry with you and record your reactions to things as they occur. For example, after a workout, write down how you feel immediately afterward. You don't need to write a lot. A dated entry can be as simple as, "Just finished 30 minutes of weight training followed by 30 minutes of jogging on the treadmill. Felt great after weight training but jogging really made my knees ache and it was difficult to get through 30 minutes."

If you feel good post-workout, these written feelings can be used to motivate you to work out on another day when you just don't feel like it (and there WILL be those days). If, however, you notice a negative trend and find that you are feeling negative emotions after your workouts or after certain meals – whether these emotions are frustration, pain, disappointment, annoyance, etc. – you will need to explore these further. It may be that your workouts or certain meals aren't suited for you and you need to be doing some other kind of activity or eating other foods that are better attuned to your interests and your body.

By documenting your reactions to the elements of your weight-loss program, you are actually doing two things: 1) distracting yourself from your impatience by focusing your attention on other things, and 2) introspecting, or taking a detailed mental examination of your thoughts and feelings. Introspection brings greater self-awareness and greater self-awareness fosters the ability to work your weight-loss program in ways that resonate with you, allowing you to make lasting changes that stick

It's like a 2-point conversion in football! *SCORE!*

DAY 10: The Tortoise and the Hare

**MOOD INDICATOR: Feeling the
need for variety…which is, after all,
the spice of life**

We all know Aesop's fable about the tortoise and the
hare. In the story, the tortoise, after being ridiculed by
the hare for his slowness, challenges the hare to a race.
The hare, confident of winning, takes time during the
race to eat, to chat with people, and to even take a nap.
The tortoise, on the other hand, plods along
methodically and ends up crossing the finish line
before the hare.

As with many of Aesop's fables, the true moral
message of this fable is left open to interpretation.
When I consider the story in the context of health and
wellness, however, I think the message is quite clear:

CONSISTENCY IS KEY!

The reason so many of us abandon our weight-loss

efforts before they come to fruition is because, all too often, we neglect a crucial part of forming long-term habits and changing behavior: consistency. We might stick to our meal and workout plans during Week 1…eating well Monday-Friday and working out 3 nights that week. But then comes the weekend.

Ah, the weekend!

Something about the weekend lures so many of us off course. Come Friday night, we, like the hare, think, "I did so good all week! I am ahead of the game and deserve to break bread and toast with my friends! What's one night of celebration going to hurt?"

Friday bleeds into Saturday (after all, it IS still the weekend… "and it would be rude NOT to take a piece of the birthday cake…I'll make up for it tomorrow…").

Next thing you know, Saturday morphs into Sunday, and the free-for-all continues.

That cheat meal we may have proactively added to our meal plan to prevent a Culinary Panic Attack (see Day 2) has suddenly turned into a cheat festival.

It's not until Monday morning that we realize we've lost ground in our overall progress toward the finish line, and then what do we do? We instinctively crank it up, trying to make up for lost time. This creates extra pressure and stress, and often comes with a dose of self-condemnation, followed by rationalization along the lines of "but it's OK – it was only this one time. I'll be back on track after this week!"

We do well Monday, Tuesday, Wednesday and even Thursday but come Friday...the cycle repeats itself.

By the third or fourth week of yo-yo'ing between consistency and inconsistency – between channeling the tortoise and then channeling the hare – most of us grow tired of the schizophrenia, rationalize that we aren't seeing progress anyway, and decide it's not worth the trouble.

What we fail to recognize is that, in order to see progress, we need to be consistent in our behaviors and mindset for at least a 30-day period. In fact, when it comes to changing the body, a common guideline states that it takes four weeks for you to notice changes in your body, eight weeks for family/friends to notice changes, and 12 weeks for everyone else to notice. So it appears that there is also a correlation between the duration of consistency and the degree of noticeable change.

Consistency isn't always fun and it's certainly not

glamorous. Just like a tortoise, consistency can be kind of boring...and maybe even a little ugly! However, if you have goals to achieve and are serious about reaching the finish line, consistency is required for success.

That said, this doesn't mean you have to stop enjoying life. However, you will likely need to plan ahead for challenging situations and find creative ways of _being as consistent as possible_ given other aspects of your life and lifestyle.

MINDSET TOOL:

Let's say you have a party or other social event coming up this month and you know that food temptations will abound. The hare is shouting, "YEEEEEESSSS! Variety at last!"

But the tortoise is repeating in a calm, steady voice, "Remember consistency, my friend...consistency."

Rather than sit back and let the party happen to you, then blame it for totally disrupting your progress, you have to be proactive and have a plan for how YOU will approach the party.

YOU ARE IN THE DRIVER'S SEAT.

I can't emphasize that enough.

But being the driver comes with responsibilities, one of which is to steer yourself safely through troubled waters. When you know a special event is approaching, perhaps you need to preemptively plan to have your cheat meal on that day and skip it on the scheduled cheat meal day. Or perhaps you need to work with your nutrition professional to tighten your eating in other ways before and/or after the special event so that you can compensate for the extra indulgence. Or maybe you don't indulge at all but just eat your regularly planned healthy foods and drink water before attending the event, then spend your time socializing instead of eating. Be creative but figure out an approach that works for you and do enough planning to ensure that the event doesn't ruin your overall consistency.

DAY 11: Acceptance and Surrender

MOOD INDICATOR: Feeling confused about all this "self-love" business

You read a lot these days about "loving yourself" and having a positive self-image no matter what you look like...and that's all well and good but what happens if you just don't naturally feel this kind of self-love? How do you plant the seeds, then nurture them and make them grow?

The first step in developing a healthy body image and creating a foundation for self-love is to practice acceptance and surrender.

According to Wikipedia, in human psychology, acceptance is "a person's assent to the reality of a situation, recognizing a process or condition (often a negative or uncomfortable situation) without attempting to change it, protest, or exit."

Prior to committing to a weight-loss program, you had to demonstrate acceptance. You had to have that moment of reckoning when you acknowledged that your well-being was in need of improvement and that your weight was not where you wanted it to be. As part of the program, you set some realistic goals to change your current state of well-being but first you had to demonstrate acceptance.

The other cornerstone of self-love, surrender, is a little trickier to master.

Surrender is acceptance of what is, PLUS embracing the unknown, without fear and without any kind of need to control. In terms of body image, surrender is a willingness to trust the weight-loss process and allow your body to transform into the best it can be without pressure to conform to predisposed notions about an "ideal" body image. It means no longer trying to force your body image to fit into any kind of mold. It means letting go of whatever image you have had in your head that has prevented you from looking in the mirror and loving your body every single day, despite its current areas for improvement or imperfections and despite the extra pounds it may be carrying. And it means replacing your current body image with a new one that honors the beauty that exists even in the presence of the things you are working to change.

Far too often, when we pass the stage of acceptance, we get derailed and become obsessed with our flaws and shortcomings and can never get to the stage of surrender. The key to surrender is the realization that the body image we may have been carrying in our heads may not even be realistic for *anyone* to achieve, never mind someone of our age, height, body frame, etc. Years of being bombarded with unrealistic media images of airbrushed models and images of celebrities who have invested in more cosmetic surgery, personal trainers and personal chefs than our pocketbooks will ever be able to afford have, both consciously and subconsciously, impacted the body image we have put on a pedestal in our Minds. Surrender involves taking down the pedestal. In so doing, we are freeing ourselves to look in the mirror and realize that the reflection staring back isn't the hideous, horrendous image we feared. In fact, it's a person who's beautiful not only in spite of but because of the imperfections…for it is truly those imperfections that make us real…that make us unique…and that are part of our story.

While it's certainly OK to want to lose weight and shed pounds, it's important not to direct negative energy toward yourself in the process. The sooner you can begin building a positive self-image even before the pounds have been lost, the sooner you will find your mindset shifting in ways that will fuel your motivation and move you closer to the achievement of your wellness goals.

> **"The marksman hitteth the mark partly by pulling, partly by letting go."**
> **~ Egyptian proverb**

In order to make changes to your physique, you have to make the effort and do some hard work – this is true – but you also have to accept and love yourself in order for sustainable transformations to occur.

MINDSET TOOL:

The next time you walk outside, pay close attention to nature. Notice the flowers, trees, leaves, grass…whatever catches your eye and take a moment to realize that none of these things are perfect. A beautiful flower may have a petal that was partially eaten by a bug but in its entirety, is it any less beautiful? A gorgeous red oak may tower overhead but when you look closely, you may see that many of its branches are dead despite the many others that are thriving. Now, if YOU were walking around with dead limbs, you'd think you were the most horrific sight to behold but here is this tree, no less majestic because of its shortcomings!

Nature is a prime example of perfection defined by a sea of imperfections. Use it as a daily reminder to embrace your own imperfections and love yourself, flaws and all.

DAY 12: Discipline vs. Willpower

MOOD INDICATOR: Feeling yourself dig your heels in the ground with an inner voice screaming, "I don't wanna! I don't wanna!"

We frequently hear the words "discipline" and "willpower" tossed around when people talk about changing existing habits and adopting a new lifestyle. In fact, the two words are often used interchangeably.

In the world of weight loss, however, discipline and willpower are not synonymous and focusing on one instead of the other (even subconsciously) is a surefire way to derail your long-term weight-loss plans. It's important to understand their differences so you know when to rely on one vs. the other.

Willpower is the strength of will to carry out one's decisions, wishes or plans, and the underlying implication is that when one exhibits willpower, one exhibits control. I tend to picture willpower as a firm, ironclad grip that one uses to manhandle cravings and other perceived weaknesses and bend them into compliance.

Willpower is tough stuff!

Discipline, on the other hand, stems historically from the idea of using systematic instruction to train a person – as in "teaching someone a discipline" – and for that reason, it has a softer connotation than willpower.

Use of the word discipline has evolved since the early days and is now used to mean an assertion of willpower over base desires, so there *is* a component of willpower inherent in discipline. However, demonstrating discipline also implies the use of reason to determine the best course of action to oppose such desires, and that's where discipline and willpower have distinct differences.

Willpower, as a more primal instinct, gives us the conviction to get started. It pushes our butts outta the gate and challenges us to reel in some of the more "base desires" that we may have allowed to go unchecked for too long.

But here's the catch: Willpower may sustain us for 10, 20, or even 30 days but ultimately we need more than the iron fist to keep us motivated.

Discipline enables us to sustain our motivation because it forces us to apply reason to our decisions and ensures alignment between what we know on an intellectual plane, with what we feel on an emotional plane, with what we do on a physical plane.

As you work through your weight-loss program, be aware of the differences between discipline and willpower. On days when you are less motivated, before you simply force yourself to do something you may not feel like doing (i.e., before you call on willpower), I encourage you first to hit pause and examine the situation a little more deeply. Intellectually, you may know that you should be doing whatever it is that's on your plan – for example, walking or drinking your water or eating consistent meals and snacks – but something in you is fighting it tooth and nail and causing the voices in your head to scream, "I don't wanna! I don't wanna!"

When you first begin forming healthy habits, you may, in fact, need to call on some willpower to just push yourself over the hump of fear and insecurity. Then all will be well. But if you're well into your program and you're experiencing this kind of internal resistance, you may need to stop and do some introspection. Discipline flows easily and effortlessly when there is alignment between the Mind (what we know intellectually we should be doing), the Spirit (what we emotionally want to do for ourselves), and the Body (what our body needs us to do for it). If we try to "willpower our way" through the times when discipline may not be flowing, it MIGHT work in the beginning, but eventually the tension between Mind/Spirit/Body will win and we'll likely just quit whatever it is we were trying to do without having the benefit of understanding what's really going on. When faced with inner conflict, it's always best to take time to introspect and ferret out the root causes.

MINDSET TOOL:

One of the most important things to do when faced with resistance during your weight-loss program is to determine the source of the resistance. More specifically, what is it that you are afraid of, because fear often breeds resistance? Fear of change is a big factor in the beginning of your journey and can be, as I already mentioned, put in check by willpower in the early stages of change. Unfortunately though, fear never really goes away. We always have to contend with it and whenever our self-discipline has been upset, it's usually because fear has slid its way into our conscious Mind. So the questions you need to ask yourself are, "What am I emotionally fearing? Why is my heart not in this right now? What do I need to do to become more emotionally clear about this and how can I realign my Mind/Spirit/Body?"

Once you understand why you are afraid, you can take action to address the root causes of the fear and realign your mindset. This realignment will automatically allow discipline to flow easily and enable you to once again work in harmony with your weight-loss program. It will also help you sustain your healthy habits long after your weight-loss program is over.

If you find that you just can't get "there"...that emotionally, you just can't connect with a certain habit or goal no matter how much introspection you do...then you may need to go back one step further and reassess or possibly revise the habit or goal itself. It's more likely though that by applying reason and challenging your fears, you can realign yourself and allow your self-discipline to keep you on track with your plan.

DAY 13: Cancel-Clear!

MOOD INDICATOR: Feeling negative and worrying about S*T*U*F*F

A few years ago, I became very interested in metaphysics and took several classes, both in-person and online. One of the coolest "tricks" I learned was how to "Cancel-Clear" negative thoughts.

The technique was so simple.

Whenever a negative thought or worry crossed my Mind, I firmly repeated in my head the words "CANCEL-CLEAR!"

Simple as that.

The theory is that by saying those words, you alert the Universe to ignore those negative thoughts and to disallow them from manifesting into form.

Different teachers presented this exercise in slightly different ways to me. Some said that repeating the words alone was enough. Others encouraged me to visualize a violet flame (associated with St. Germain) consuming the negative thoughts and sweeping them away.

At that time, I was doing a lot of worrying. I was working for a bankrupt company and felt constant pressure about job security. Trying something as simple as saying "Cancel-Clear" every time a worry about my job or money arose seemed easy enough to give a try.

Surprisingly, the tactic worked wonders and put a lot of anxiety at bay. When I began to practice it, I also added an element of "letting go" to the exercise by releasing to a Higher Power all the things about which I was worrying…things outside of my control. So in essence, I was cancelling/clearing my own "oops" in thinking and then sealing it with a blanket of faith and trust that everything was going to be OK.

I later emailed my sister about doing this when she was having so much anxiety that she couldn't sleep at night. You don't know my sister but suffice it to say that she doesn't take the same experimental approach to life that I do, so for her to even try this technique was surprising. Even more surprising, however, was that she, too, found it to be extremely helpful in reducing her levels of stress and worry.

Don't always assume everything in life has to be complicated. Often the simple things have the greatest influence because they are easy to do and quickly turn into habits.

MINDSET TOOL:

Just as the phrase "Cancel-Clear" can be used to clear negative thoughts in general, I believe similar "thought-sweeping" phrases can be used to clear the Mind when the subconscious allows negative things to creep in about our body image or our ability to stick with a weight-loss program. To incorporate this secret weapon into your arsenal, first name at least one thing about yourself/your body that you like…or, better yet, LOVE! For example, let's say you have a great smile. The next time you find yourself being overly critical of yourself/your body…thinking things like, "My thighs are so flabby!" or "My hips are just getting wider and wider!" or "I can't possibly wear THAT! I'll look like a pig stuffed in a poke!" (←OK, that last one is one of mine!!!)…stop the thought immediately and replace it with something like, "Yeah, OK…so what? I still have the best and most contagious smile in the entire city…maybe even the state! And that's what people notice and remember…not my stupid thighs!"

Make it fun!

Taunt yourself! I often talk back to my Negative Mind and say things like, "Oh yeah, Buddy?!" to let it know who's in charge!

Exaggerate! Maybe you don't think you REALLY have the best smile in the city but no one is going to hold court on this. For just this once, shut down the Analytical Mind. Go with the flow and use whatever statement your Positive Mind gives you…then see how quickly the self-doubt and self-defeating thought patterns go slithering back into the crevices from which they came!!!

DAY 14: It's All About the Swag!
MOOD INDICATOR: Feeling
insecure

Usually I pass by "before" and "after" transformation photos without giving them much notice because the skeptic in me questions the validity of the results vs. the power of lighting and the perfect camera angle. The other day, however, I noticed some "before" and "after" body transformations online that actually caught my attention. These photos were unusual because they didn't depict dramatic physical changes. Sure, I could see some obvious changes in the subject's physique: her face was thinner, her legs were leaner, and her abs were definitely cut. But what struck me more than her physical transformation was the change in how she was carrying herself.

At first glance, her stance might have looked identical in each photo but if you looked more closely at the "after" shot, her shoulders were less slumped, her hands were higher on her hips, her hair was more relaxed…and she was smiling!

In short, the "after" shot reflected CONFIDENCE…and it suddenly occurred to me:

It's all about the swag.

In fact, when I examined this girl's features even more closely and looked at her basic shape, her face, etc., I also realized that she's quite ordinary. And yet, because of her confidence…because of how she carries herself…she has found her way into the hearts of the millions who see her in a popular at-home workout program.

You don't have to be one of America's top models to be seen as beautiful and win the admiration of others. Loving yourself, taking care of yourself, being proud of yourself…those are the things that will shine from the inside out and draw others to you. And often it's not physical appearance that wins admirers. It's the respect you have for yourself that makes other stop and pay attention, too.

MINDSET TOOL:

As you begin to feel more comfortable in your skin over the course of your weight-loss journey, I want you to play with "swag." The next time you are walking down the halls at work or in a store or in any public place, push your shoulders back a little more than normal, lift your chin a little higher, mentally tell yourself "I'm awesome – I ROCK!" and see how it feels.

Notice how others respond.

You are putting some hard work into your program – you have every right to flaunt it. My bet is that in doing so, you'll boost your self-confidence and others will detect and respond to that. All of this will, in turn, fuel your motivation for continued healthy living and further solidify the healthy habits you're adopting.

DAY 15: Tapping Into Your Intuition

**MOOD INDICATOR: Feeling stable
and clear but open to new ideas**

Western civilization has trained us to honor the analytical Brain and glorify the power of thinking. The concept of Mind-Body connection is becoming mainstream these days and while that is a huge step in the right direction for the collective consciousness, focusing on the Mind-Body alone leaves out an important "catch."

Not only do we need to reconnect the Mind and Body but we have to get the Brain out of the way, too!

Although analysis and thinking certainly have their place in the world, an important part of healthy living is learning how to balance the Brain's influence in the Mind-Body equation. The way to do this is by developing Intuition.

Simply put, Intuition is a way of knowing, oftentimes felt right down in our gut – in the very core of our being – and oftentimes without any rational reason FOR knowing. As it applies to wellness, Intuition is the feeling we get that draws us toward healthy foods instead of less healthy alternatives or the feeling that we need to stick with our wellness plan even when temptations may be luring us off course. It's a general sense of knowing what's best for our bodies that prompts us to follow through with actions that support those best interests.

Have you ever watched a dog sniff a treat before he decides to eat it? On some level, he's determining with his nose if it will be tasty, and, if he's especially particular like my dog, if it's worth his time! But on another level, I truly believe he is using his instincts/intuition (aided by his sense of smell) to determine whether the food placed before him is safe and desirable.

There will be times during your weight-loss journey when something doesn't sit right and you find yourself getting into an internal debate about something included in your plan. Maybe it's the fact that your plan allows unlimited quantities of artificial sweeteners that are zero-calorie and have no impact on insulin levels (i.e., stevia, monk fruit, etc.). Intellectually, the

Brain agrees with your plan and argues that this has scientifically been proven not to impact weight in controlled studies. But something tells you this isn't working for you...that you feel like you're retaining water or just not feeling like you're at your best after you chug a zero-calorie "sports drink."

Tell the Brain to get out of your way!

Just because it's in your plan and just because the Brain says it's technically OK doesn't mean you HAVE to do it, especially if your Intuition is telling you otherwise.

Part of being healthy means being mindful. Mindfulness means paying attention to the moment and how you feel in that moment.

Like the dog that sniffs the highly processed kibbles and walks away, even though that's all his owner put in his bowl, you, too, should turn away from anything in your plan that your Intuition tells you doesn't resonate with your body. If you're working with a professional, talk to him/her about your concerns and reluctance. If he/she tells you there is no other way but the plan you were delivered (and I have been told this by a so-called professional), find another person to help you. If you're working on your own, research your options and find substitutes to replace the things that set off your Intuition's alarm system (for example, try water with fresh fruit slices to replace artificially-sweetened sports drinks).

MINDSET TOOL:

The more we allow our Intuition to have a voice, the more developed it becomes and the more it can help us. Here are a few exercises you can try to develop your Intuition into a strong tool that you may use beyond just your weight-loss journey:

Take time every day to listen to your body.

The shower is an ideal place to do this because you typically have at least a few minutes of total down time, just standing there with water streaming over your head. In those few minutes, do a full-body scan with your Mind. Start at your head and visually work your way down your body, visualizing negative energy flowing out of your feet and down the drain with the water. As you perform the scan, pay attention to any odd feelings or things you may notice. You may or may not detect anything the first few times you do this exercise but as you practice, you may find that you become adept at noticing energy blockages (often aligned with areas of physical pain) or just things that need extra tender loving care.

Consider keeping a dream journal to capture any intuitive moments that occur during your sleep.

You might even want to ask your Intuitive Self a question before bedtime and see if any answers come through while you sleep. It may take a few tries but something may eventually come through that can help you. Also, once you begin recording your dreams, it seems that 1) you dream more frequently and 2) the ability to remember your dreams improves. It's as though the Universe rewards you for working with the tools it provides by making the tools even more powerful as you go. (And from my own experience, dream journals can continue to provide insight when you read them again years later; sometimes they provide a healthy dose of comedy and entertainment, too!).

Meditate.

Meditation is a GREAT way to get in touch with and build Intuition. If you have trouble quieting the chattering monkeys in your head, consider downloading guided meditations from iTunes or other websites and use them to develop your own meditation practice.

DAY 16: Sometimes It's Just a Matter of Science

MOOD INDICATOR: Feeling confused and frustrated by the number on the scale

I promised in the Introduction that I wouldn't get into the mind-boggling science behind weight loss and nutrition but I have to make one small exception in order to prevent you from being discouraged by a certain type of weight-loss plateau that you are bound to hit. I will keep it really simple. Just bear with me and then I'll get back to addressing the mental game and explain why the scientific explanation is important.

After about three weeks of following a weight-loss program, many of you will hit what is known as a weight-loss plateau. Up to this point, you have been watching the number on the scale drop with some degree of regularity. Then suddenly, at no fault of your own, the number stops changing. You haven't deviated from your scheduled meals or workouts, so what's going on?

Take a nice deep breath and relax. Despite the stagnation that appears to be happening on the surface, something really awesome may be happening behind the scenes. In order to lose fat, the body must burn it as energy. In order to burn it as energy, the body has to combine the body fat with oxygen to make carbon dioxide and water. Carbon dioxide and water are heavier than fat because of the oxygen that is added to create them. Although the carbon dioxide is released fairly quickly (in the process of breathing), it may take the body longer to get rid of the water, which first must pass into the spaces between cells then into the bloodstream, on to the kidneys, and finally to the bladder for excretion. In essence, the plateau you may experience, especially around Week 3, may simply be some water weight that your body hasn't yet been able to expel. You will likely notice an increase in urination when your body has finally been able to "catch up" and release the excess water, and that's also when your plateau should break.

In addition to the Week 3 plateau, you may also notice after the first few weeks that your weight may fluctuate by as much as three pounds from one day to the next. It's hard to believe that's possible but it is, and the reason is because of hydration and water balance. You may still be losing 1-2 pounds of body fat but that fat loss may be masked by the water-weight fluctuations, so don't despair!

MINDSET TOOL:

Water is retained based on the sodium in our diets, our body's response to the foods we're consuming, hormone levels, and a laundry list of other factors, so it's sometimes hard to tell what may be triggering weight fluctuations. The best thing you can do is keep notes throughout your weight-loss journey. Record the things you eat (including cheats; honesty is key here!) and the reflection that those things have on the scale. For example, if you ate dinner, which included a ½ cup of brown rice, at 9 PM one night, and you weighed 2 pounds more in the morning, your body may not respond well to carbohydrates in the evening. One night/morning is, of course, not enough data to confirm this suspicion but if you keep consistent notes, you can begin to see patterns and piece together the puzzle.

Document the types of workouts you do each day and see if that plays a role. Some people report that doing too much cardio causes them to retain water. For me, plyometrics trigger weight gain (and, in my case, I can assure you it's not muscle – it's water).

Ladies, record how changes (or lack of changes) on the scale correlate to certain days in your menstrual cycle.

Become your own detective and over time, you'll begin to understand your body so well that you may even come to anticipate weight fluctuations before stepping on the scale.

No matter what you do: STAY THE COURSE!

Do not despair and revert back to your former eating and exercise habits if you see wonky things happening on the scale. Sometimes the weight-loss plateau or weight gain that you experience is purely about science and the only thing you can do is be patient and do your detective work. Panicking or berating yourself for pounds that may not even be your "fault" will only increase your stress levels and potentially raise your cortisol (and we all know that stress-induced cortisol is usually not our friend). If you're up against what may be a water-induced plateau, give the process some time (at least a week) and then make an assessment about next steps. By then, the plateau may break. If it doesn't and you're working with a professional, ask his/her opinion and see if your plan may be due for some tweaking. If you're working alone, go back to your online resources and use your notes to see if your plan may benefit from some adjustments.

I like to keep weight loss as simple as possible but I think there is some comfort in at least understanding that the human body is a complex machine. Things don't always happen in a linear fashion the way we'd like them to happen and if we simply remember that and wait out the natural processes without worrying or becoming upset, we may be pleasantly surprised at what our bodies ultimately can do.

DAY 17: Help! I'm Being Sabotaged!

MOOD INDICATOR: Feeling
frustrated with family members (or
yourself!)

Scenario #1:

It's happened yet again. You walk in the door to find a bag of potato chips wide open on your kitchen counter, staring you smack in the face, while the tub of French onion dip looks on with what you would swear is a smirk, if only inanimate objects had smirking abilities.

You try to look away.

You don't even like chips all that much but something about the taste of salt and the mere fact that you know this is "forbidden food" seems to be drawing you in and overtaking all rational thought.

Amidst the waves of temptation, you feel anger surging through your body. You've asked your kids time and time again to keep that crap out of sight. You sat them down and talked to them about what you're trying to accomplish and why, and the reason it's so important to you. They nodded their heads in understanding and fed you some platitudes that made you think they were on board but this has to be the fifth or sixth time you've come home to a buffet of temptations strewn across the counter to test your mettle and resolve. And your spouse has been no better, making microwave popcorn for a TV-watching snack every night (it's TV, for Pete's sake! Not the movie theater!).

Scenario #2:

Maybe you don't have kids and it was YOU who left that bag on the counter, not opened with dip alongside but sitting out in plain sight (sometimes, that can be just as brutal). You knew better. You knew you should have thrown it away when your friend brought it over the other night, but instead you let it sit there and now it's taunting you in its colorful packaging (packaging that you just know some highly-compensated marketing person designed based on its ability to trigger insane cravings and emotional eating. That heartless bastard.).

While it's understandable to be frustrated when family

members do things that make it more difficult to stick to your weight-loss program, or when you yourself are the cause of unnecessary temptation, I'm about to give you a healthy dose of tough love that applies to either scenario.

Ready?

You are the one who chose to take this weight-loss journey.

YOU.

Not your kids. Not your spouse or partner. Not your mother or your father or the sweet neighbor who keeps bringing over baked goods for no apparent reason other than she has a lot of time on her hands and no immediate family with whom to share her treats.

Ideally, you have a strong support system in place for your weight-loss journey. You're surrounded by family and friends who know what you're trying to achieve and who are willing to do what they can to offer emotional support along the way. But even in an ideal world, unless your entire support system happens to be following the exact same weight-loss program as you, and also happens to be going through every emotional up and down as you, no support system is going to be 100% perfect, 100% of the time. That's just not feasible.

The cold hard truth is that YOU chose to make changes in YOUR lifestyle, but they did not choose to make changes in theirs. While it's fair to ask that they emotionally support you and that they don't sabotage your progress by pressuring you to eat foods excluded from your plan, it's another to expect them to alter all of their behaviors on your behalf. There has to be some "give and take." It would be nice if your kids and spouse or partner could remember to put away their snacks so that you aren't greeted by a bag of chips taunting you, but if they forget, you have to remember that this is not their priority nor is it their journey. It's yours. And to that end, you have to be the one to take greater responsibility and exhibit greater discipline.

It's also not realistic to expect that you won't be faced with temptations that you yourself create. You can't protect yourself from everything in the world that may tempt you. You simply need to remember that no one is forcing you to do this. You chose to start this journey and you can choose to end it as well. By simply giving this some consideration, you will likely diffuse the feelings of anger, mentally recommit to your goals, calmly put away the chips and dip, and move on.

MINDSET TOOL:

If you have not already done so, I encourage you to reorganize your kitchen. Dedicate specific cupboards/shelf space for your food and other cupboards/shelf space for the rest of the family. Do the same thing in the refrigerator, giving yourself specific refrigerator shelves (preferably those at eye level) and drawer space for your food.

When you are craving food, go only to the places you know are dedicated to you.

If it helps, label your food and your food storage areas.

Use sticky notes or other labels to clearly denote food that's included in your meal plan. These notes act as reminders not only for your family but also for you. Seeing a shelf labeled "Family" and one labeled "My Stuff" will, at a minimum, force you to think about your food choices and hopefully drive you toward the right shelf. It may also remind family members to return foods to the appropriate shelves when they are done eating.

You can also label particularly tempting foods to remind yourself to either avoid or eat them in moderation. For example, my husband has a peanut butter addiction and eats a jar of natural peanut butter every week (I kid you not). I, too, love peanut butter but don't have the ability to metabolize it the way he does so, in order to control my temptation to overindulge, I put a sticky note on the jar that says "DALE – DON'T GO OVERBOARD! EAT IN MODERATION!" Using my name on the note makes it even harder to ignore.

While they may sound silly, these tools really DO work. However, effectiveness aside and for argument's sake, even if they ARE silly, who's going to judge you? Chances are your refrigerator and cupboards are viewed by a limited audience and there's really no one you need to impress.

If you're committed to losing weight, you must be willing to do what it takes to help yourself stay on the Weight Loss Wagon and that may very well mean checking your ego at the station before you board!

DAY 18: The Importance of Packaging

MOOD INDICATOR: Feeling stable
but wanting to avoid future temptation

Who doesn't love to receive a gift, especially when it's wrapped in pretty paper and garnished with a ribbon and bow? The entire process of receiving a gift is ALL ABOUT YOU and is designed to make you feel special. How can you NOT enjoy that?

Unfortunately, the age of impersonal gift cards and the even more detached *electronic* gift cards has nearly made the art of personalized gift giving and gift wrapping a thing of the past. You can, however, use the distant memory of the last time you received a gift embellished in the finest couture and apply those same principles to your weight-loss program.

When we think about weight loss and our five senses, we naturally think first about the senses of taste and smell since those are most readily associated with food.

However, we do have three other senses from which the Brain receives signals and I would argue that one of those, vision, plays as strong a role (if not stronger) as taste and smell.

At times, looks might be everything when it comes to sticking with your weight-loss program.

The looks of your food, that is.

What on earth am I talking about, you ask? Allow me to explain by indulging me in a visualization exercise.

Let's presume you like oatmeal (if you don't, substitute another hot cereal of choice into this exercise). Close your eyes and picture a serving of oatmeal in a bowl you've had for 10+ years and that you bought during a difficult time in your life. The bowl is sitting on the kitchen counter with a spoon beside it because you usually eat it right there, standing up in the kitchen, in an effort to save a few precious minutes of time as you rush to get to work. The cereal sits in a clump at the bottom of the bowl but a trail of cereal leads up to the rim because of your sloppy and hurried serving. Cinnamon is dumped in a small pile in the center and hot steam is coming off the top.

Open your eyes.

While the cinnamon and hot steam may have had some appeal, chances are that you winced a little at the rest of the scene. Instead of seeing a soothing, warm, comfort food, you saw instead a lumpy dollop of bland cereal sitting in the middle of a gloomy old bowl, waiting to be hastily eaten in a mad rush to get out the door to work.

Clear the image from your memory.

Now close your eyes again but this time picture a serving of oatmeal in a brand new bowl of your favorite color (or, better yet, in a blue bowl, since eating off blue dishes has been shown to make us eat less). The bowl is sitting on a clean placemat (again of your favorite color…or blue!) on your kitchen table with a napkin beside it. A shiny new spoon is delicately placed to one side of the bowl, ready to be picked up and used. Cinnamon is sprinkled across the entire bowl with a light coating of natural sweetener and some small chunks of real apple added as extra garnish. Hot steam is waving off the top of the cereal, wafting the smell of warm cinnamon into the air.

Open your eyes.

Do you see how the presentation of your food and the visual experience can make a difference in your mental attitude? Essentially the same breakfast (oatmeal) was transformed from an ugly, unappealing dollop into a much more tempting comfort food simply by virtue of its presentation.

MINDSET TOOL:

While I recognize that you won't likely have time to make EVERY meal or snack appeal to your visual senses, I want you to understand how important visual display can be and use it in your favor whenever possible. If you hate drinking water but know you're supposed to increase your intake for weight loss, try pouring what may otherwise seem like boring water into a wine glass or even a champagne flute, drop a couple slices of lemon, lime, watermelon or cucumber into it, and voila! That boring water may have just transformed into something that not only appeals to your sense of sight but also attracts your taste buds a little more as well.

Think about some of the foods on your plan that you don't really like all that much. Then think of ways that you can garnish them or present them to make them more appealing.

And if you're using a set of dishes you used during a particularly bad time in your life, for heaven's sake, stop doing that!

Our association with things can be extremely influential and you don't want negative associations with your set of dishes to tarnish the positive associations you are trying to make with your new eating habits and foods.

Another way to leverage your sense of sight on your weight-loss journey is to gift wrap some of your food items. If you have certain foods in your eating plan that you're only allowed to eat on certain days (maybe these are cheat days or maybe these are just foods you don't get every day of the week but you really like and would be tempted to eat every day if you could), portion them out and wrap the appropriate serving sizes in small packages in the refrigerator. Make them actual gifts! You can easily put wrapping paper around a storage container, don it with a ribbon and bow, and then add a tag with your name on it. Every time you wander into the kitchen and open the refrigerator (which usually happens when you are not supposed to be eating anything in the first place), that little gift serves as a visual reminder that a present is waiting for you if you just keep on track. Plus, it's less tempting to binge or cheat when you have to go through the process of unwrapping foods that you yourself put extra care into wrapping.

Weight loss is a mental game, people!

You might think some of this stuff is outright crazy but as Albert Einstein once said, "You have to learn the rules of the game. And then you have to play better than anyone else." Learning to play better than anyone else means understanding yourself and learning the tricks that will help you play to win. If wrapping your food in the refrigerator helps teach you how to control cravings, then do it. Once you learn the art of self-control, you may not need to wrap any more food but don't be ashamed to use the tool to get yourself started.

On the weight-loss journey, it is imperative that you check your ego at the door. This isn't about pride. This is about building self-awareness and doing things to create habits on which you can rely for the rest of your life.

DAY 19: In Defense of Setting Boundaries and Acting With a Healthy Dose of Selfishness

MOOD INDICATOR: Feeling guilty

To a large extent, your success with weight loss will depend on your ability to say "no" without feeling guilty.

I was raised in the Roman Catholic Church and by parents who'd lived through the Great Depression. "Guilt" and "Self-Sacrifice" (particularly for the betterment of other family members) may as well have been my middle names. These were two qualities that my upbringing strongly instilled in me.

So when I hear people, especially women, talk about how difficult it is to do things for themselves, like work out or make healthy meals, because of their obligations to other people (spouses, partners, children, parents, friends, the list goes on), I get it. I really do get it.

Living my life with what I call "a healthy dose of selfishness" was not something I was born doing. In fact, it took me the better part of 35 years and relationships with not one or two but several self-absorbed, narcissistic boyfriends who "took" far more than they "gave" for me to figure this out. I could write another book on how those relationships helped me master the art of healthy selfishness but for our purposes here, please take my word for it – I know the challenge of mastering this art!

In terms of the success of your weight-loss journey, selfishness is not only desirable – it's required. To maintain long-term, sustainable results, you have to learn to put guilt on the shelf and accept the fact that selfishness in this context is healthy and beneficial.

It will fuel your motivation and maintain your commitment to the things you set out to do. It will keep your eye on the target, even when things are going madcap crazy around you, and it will enable you to remain true to your priorities.

And when you take a step back and look objectively at your current situation…isn't a lack of selfishness what got you here in the first place? Think about it. Think

about all the times you skipped the gym because you
had to cart the kids to sports practice. All the times you
made your husband the meat-and-potatoes dinner he
wanted, leaving no time to make the fish and
vegetables that YOU wanted to make for yourself. All
the times you attended social events where you felt
peer-pressured to eat and drink things you knew
weren't healthy for you because you didn't want to
insult the host or hostess. If you'd been putting
yourself first and tending to your needs instead of
everyone else's, it's highly possible those extra pounds
wouldn't have crept up on you and you wouldn't be
back on the Weight Loss Wagon.

**Insanity is said to be doing the same thing over
and over and expecting different results.**

If lack of selfishness has led you to where you are
today, isn't it time you tried something else on for size?

Now before you get all anxious on me and begin to fret
that I'm asking you to totally upset the dynamics of
your household or social circles, let me be very clear. In
no way am I proposing that you abandon your
responsibilities as a parent, spouse, partner, friend, etc.
That's what's cool about acting with a *healthy* dose of
selfishness. It's not over the top. You aren't going to

turn into a Queen B because all of a sudden, it's all about you. What you ARE going to do is re-establish your priorities and make your weight-loss program one of them.

You're probably thinking, "Wait. Wasn't that what I did when I began this journey – made weight loss a priority?"

No, not really. What you did was take an important first step. You set goals, sought out resources, and decided on the eating and exercise plans you'd follow. You boarded the Weight Loss Wagon. But just because you boarded doesn't mean you actually put weight loss at the top of your list of priorities. And even if you did, once life started happening all around you, it's quite possible your priorities got shuffled and your focus got blurry.

MINDSET TOOL:

Right now, this very minute, I want you to take out a sheet of paper and jot down your personal priorities in rank order. If your health/weight loss is not somewhere at the top, you may need to evaluate your reasons for taking this journey and potentially put it on hold until you're ready to make it a priority.

Yes, it's that serious.

I am willing to bet that many of you had your
health/weight loss in the top 3 or 5 but put your
children and/or spouse/partner first. I am not here to
tell you that your priorities are wrong but I would at
least like you to consider the reality that if you are in
poor health, you won't be able to take care of them
anyway. It may feel awkward but listing yourself first
is really the best way to ensure that you are capable of
caring for everything and everyone else on your list.

Now that you have your list of priorities, think about
how your actions have been mirroring those priorities.
Have you been missing workouts because of
obligations to other people? If your health/weight loss
is a priority, this shouldn't happen. But let's say in this
case, the obligations have been to take your kids to
athletic practices. You obviously don't want to deny
them their chance to participate in sports so sometimes
you may need to figure out ways to meet their needs
but also meet your own. Perhaps you need to start
working out in the early morning hours. If your
health/weight loss is a priority, that should trump any
"I'm not a morning person" thoughts that just flashed
across your Mind. Or maybe you need to share driving
duties with your spouse, partner or another parent on
the team who happens to live near you. If you alternate
days, you've at least bought yourself a few workout

days you would have otherwise foregone.

My point is – when you make weight loss your priority, you will be inspired and find creative ways to stick to your plans. It may require better time management on your part or it may mean you get comfortable asking others for help (i.e., sharing the load and not doing everything yourself). It may also require you to say "no" on occasion and be OK with that (you don't HAVE to attend every party to which you are invited, and if you explain to the host/ess that you're following a weight-loss program and can't subject yourself to that degree of temptation yet, I am sure he/she will understand).

When your health is at stake, you're practically obligated to be selfish and for those who don't immediately understand, just remind them that a "healthy you" can do more for everyone. An "unhealthy you," on the other hand, will soon be able to help no one. Often that simple and logical reminder is all it takes to bring understanding and a stronger degree of support.

DAY 20: Breaking It Down

MOOD INDICATOR: Feeling overwhelmed and hopeless

"Mama said there'd be days like this...." and she wasn't kidding.

You're not sure how it happened. Yesterday you were on top of the world, feeling like you had your weight-loss goals in the bag and that you were going to nail the rest of your program. Today you woke up wondering how on earth you are going to choke down the meals on your plan and make it through the workout you're supposed to do.

You get out of bed to take your morning shower and catch a glimpse in the mirror. On top of the change in attitude, you would swear you also look heavier today than you did yesterday. As you step into the shower, you begin to wonder what the point of all your hard work is if you can wake up on any given day and feel completely rotten and…well…fat. You start to panic about not wanting to live the rest of your life like this, always struggling with your weight, and you feel the tears begin to well up in your eyes as the hot water beats down on your head.

At first glance, this might seem to be a simple, self-indulgent pity party. Upon closer look, however, you will discover that the scenario described above has a little more substance to it than pure self-pity. It's not merely about feeling victimized. It's about feeling overwhelmed, and during a weight-loss journey, there will be more than one day when you feel this way.

Change on any level is uncomfortable. When you change something about yourself – something personal like your weight – it can be outright disruptive. And when the Brain takes over the Mind, things can get out of hand really fast. You can go from being perfectly happy with your program and your progress to nearly hyperventilating at the thought of following your program for one more minute.

Unlike a Culinary Panic Attack, this type of panic attack isn't related to a particular food that's excluded from your plan. The anxiety related to this attack stems from the feeling that you simply can't do any more.

You're tapped out.
TILT.

MINDSET TOOL:

When a panic attack of this nature strikes, remember three words:

BREAK IT DOWN.

Sometimes when we focus on the big picture and consider everything all at once, we lose focus altogether. We simply have to take a step back and break the big picture down into bite-sized pieces and focus on one thing at a time.

If you feel as though you won't be able to stick to your eating plan for the entire day, stop worrying about the entire day. Focus on breakfast first. See if you can get through that meal in compliance with your plan. It's just one meal. You can certainly manage that and then you can worry about the next snack or meal...and the next and the next. Just take each one as it comes, one at a time, and before you know it, you'll be heading to bed, feeling like you just conquered Mount Everest for having stayed on the Weight Loss Wagon one more day.

If you're feeling certain that you won't be able to

survive today's workout, make a pact with yourself to get through the first 5 minutes. Anyone can do 5 minutes, right? Then at the 5-minute mark, see how you feel. Feeling good? Go for 5 minutes more. If you continue to use this approach, you're likely to find yourself re-energized and able to finish the entire workout, looking back on what you thought you were completely incapable of doing and wondering why you ever had your doubts!

DAY 21: Expecting vs. Believing

MOOD INDICATOR: Feeling hopeful and optimistic

Self-confidence is a cornerstone not just to weight loss but to any type of success. You have to believe in yourself in order to accomplish things.

If you sit back on your haunches thinking, "I can't, I can't, I can't," well…you won't, you won't, you won't.

It's as simple as that.

But belief is not enough. There has to be something else at work, something else that's going to drive you round the bases and bring you home with conviction.

That something is expectation.

Expectation goes beyond just believing in your abilities to achieve a goal. Expectation is the anticipation of results. Expectation means you already KNOW you're going to achieve what you set out to achieve. You're now just eagerly waiting for it to happen!

Expectation doesn't leave room for doubt or what-if scenarios. It comes from deep within your core and is that flutter of excitement you feel when you visualize yourself sashaying across a room of crowded people, not with the body you have today but with the physique you are working to obtain. It's that unwavering certainty that your continued efforts toward weight loss will, in fact, pay dividends and create for you the body you desire.

My first experience with the tremendous power of expectation was unfortunately not a good one. I was 9 or 10 years old and in a gymnastics meet. As I had done in so many meets before this one, I was sitting off to the side of the apparatus, mentally preparing for my floor routine, which was up next. As I visualized myself performing the routine, for reasons I cannot to this day explain, I pictured myself "falling out" of a move I had never before done wrong. I can still remember the experience as if it was yesterday because it was so startling. Although it had never before happened, the visualized error felt intensely real. Unfortunately, at that young age, I hadn't yet learned the mental tricks you can use to cancel-clear negative thoughts (see Day 13), and almost immediately after being jolted back to reality by the mental picture of my error, my number was called to perform my routine and away I went, starting in the center of the floor mat and going into the motions I had done countless times before.

What ultimately happened is exactly what you might expect. When I got to that part of my routine, I executed everything just as I had visualized…error and all.

Yes, I fell out of the move and was penalized for it.

Being the perfectionist that I am, I was devastated, but not so much because I had made a mistake but because I felt like I had known in advance it was coming and didn't do anything to stop it. Though that wasn't one of the happiest memories from my childhood, the lesson was invaluable. The power of the Mind and the power of expectations are not to be taken lightly.

Expectations don't just apply to special events. We carry the expectations we have for ourselves and for our personal success with us all day, every day.

If we nurture those expectations and feed them positive thoughts, they can be our allies.

If we ignore them or allow them to become tainted (as I did just before performing my gymnastics routine), they can quickly morph into our arch enemies.

As you continue your weight-loss journey, my guess is that you will want as many allies as you can find and lucky for you there are ways to shape your expectations so that they will promote your long-term success.

MINDSET TOOL:

Introducing the practice of visualization. Visualization is one of the best tools you can use to shape your expectations.

In the simplest of terms, visualization is creating a mental image or intention of what you want to happen and how you want to feel. Think of it as a mental dress rehearsal, right down to the emotions and sensations you experience as a result of the imagery (that last part is an important point and we'll come back to that in a minute).

We all know that the Mind is one sharp cookie but it's not the Brain. It doesn't know the difference between what's real and what's imagined. So when you visualize the successful accomplishment of your goals, for instance, the Mind retains the information as if it really happened. Repeated over the course of time, visualization can help you build confidence and rewire your thoughts to move you in the healthy direction you want to go.

Because visualization involves emotions, it's a great tool for building positive expectations. (Remember that expectations involve feelings of excitement and anticipation, so influencing expectations will require that you work on an emotional/feeling level.) By building positive expectations, you are adding an ally to your team and reinforcing your ability to accomplish what you set out to achieve.

If you really want to make the power of expectations work in your favor, take five minutes every day to perform a visualization exercise. Close your eyes and picture yourself doing things that support your weight-loss journey. Maybe you picture yourself ordering healthy menu options at dinner tonight if you know you're eating out and may be tempted off your plan. Or maybe you visualize yourself doing your entire cardio workout without taking any breaks. Or maybe you see yourself flaunting that new body of yours at an upcoming party you're planning to attend. Whatever it is, visualize it with as much clarity and detail as possible and pay attention to how it makes you feel. Notice the thoughts and feelings you have when the hostess of the party opens the door and says, "Oh my gosh! You look FABULOUS!" Or how you feel after you visually finish your cardio workout without taking any breaks. Make those five minutes of visualization work for you and exercise all facets of your imagination. Ideally, this exercise should be visual (focusing on images and pictures), kinesthetic (focusing on how the body feels), emotional (focusing on your mood and feelings), and auditory (focusing on the sounds around you, including the voices and comments of other people).

I know at least one of you, dear readers, is rolling your eyes and getting ready to skip to the next chapter without giving this tool a fair shot. Before you write this practice off as woo-woo though, consider that many elite athletes use this technique to prepare for competition (obviously with better success than I did as a young gymnast who didn't even realize she was formally visualizing!). A recent study at McGill University also applied the practice of visualization to weight loss and found that the best way to improve eating habits is not simply to create a healthy eating plan but to also visualize yourself following it.

How you visualize yourself is one of the greatest predictors of your weight-loss success.

DAY 22: Slow Progress Is Better Than No Progress

MOOD INDICATOR: Boy! This is taking a long time!

So here you are…weeks into your weight-loss journey…and you're pretty darned proud of yourself. You've been consistently applying your new eating habits and performing your workout routines. You weren't even tempted by the cookies and cake that your kids left out on the table or your co-workers put in the office break room.

The only problem is…the scale hasn't budged and you've ruled out a water-related plateau like the one explained on Day 16.

You're feeling plain old confused because you're doing everything "right" but not seeing the results you think you ought to be seeing by now. You've begun wondering if maybe it's just you…that maybe you're genetically predisposed to be heavier than others or maybe it's your hormones. Whatever it is, you know it's nothing you're doing or not doing because your compliance to your program has been spot-on.

First off, I don't recommend blind compliance to ANY weight-loss program, no matter who created it for you. Asking questions is always encouraged.

If you're not seeing results and you have truly been compliant for weeks on end, you're right – it's nothing you're doing/not doing in terms of compliance with your plan but you may not be following the right program to meet your goals. Remember what I said on Day 9: as much as this is a weight-loss journey, it's also an experiment and a process of trial and error. If you're working with a nutrition professional, talk to him/her about your frustrations and see if it's time to change your plan. If you're working on your own, doing the detective work I discussed on Day 9 becomes even more crucial in figuring out the right weight-loss formula for you. Maybe your meal plans are OK but you're not doing enough cardio. Maybe you're doing too much cardio and need to consider some weight training. The possible causes of stalled weight loss are endless and only good, solid data can help unravel the mystery. If you haven't been documenting this kind of information, go back to Day 9 and read about how to do that...then get started. The sooner you can start seeing patterns and possible connections, the better.

Now, let's say you've been tracking data and you feel like your program is well-structured and suited for you. If the program isn't the problem, you have to consider the old saying:

SLOW progress is better than NO progress.

I would be willing to bet money that, after several weeks of compliance with your plan, you will experience some sort of progress. It may not be seen on the scale, if that's where you're first looking. It may first begin as general FEELINGS of better health (more energy, being more comfortable in your skin, better digestion, etc.). Or maybe your clothes are starting to feel looser or your measurements are beginning to change, even in small increments. Chances are, SOMETHING is happening, so hang in there and don't give up yet! Look at the big picture and be open to seeing things beyond the number on the scale.

You are a mortal human being, and consequently, you were born with limitations. We all were.

Make sure you aren't sabotaging your own

success by striving for perfection when what you should be striving for is progress.

MINDSET TOOL:

If you haven't already done so, now may be a good time to start taking progress photos of yourself. Typically, these are done in shorts and a tank top or a bathing suit – some kind of attire that shows enough of your body to be able to show changes over time. You can set your digital camera on self-timer and take them in complete privacy. I usually have my head cut off in the photos, too, just so I am not distracted by things like my hair's desperate need for recoloring vs. changes in my body! It's best to take three photos – one each from the front, side and back. Then you can compare the three different angles with future photos. As you continue to work your plan, take progress photos on a regular basis (every week or every other week, depending on how well you're following your plan) and you may soon notice changes in yourself that are not evident on the scale.

I personally find progress photos to be an excellent tool for initiating change and also for fueling motivation throughout the weight-loss journey. Photos really do capture things to which you might otherwise be oblivious and help keep you focused.

DAY 23: Holy Smokes! I Really HAVE Established New Habits!
MOOD INDICATOR: Feeling like it's too easy

There may be times during your weight-loss program when you suddenly realize: "This feels too easy."

Things that were once a struggle and a challenge now happen without effort. Your 5 AM dalliance with the snooze button before dragging yourself out of bed and to the gym is no more. Now you just pop up at the first sound, sometimes feeling eager and excited to hurry up and get your workout started! Doing your weekly food prep is no longer a dreaded chore but something to which you look forward, especially since you've been experimenting with spices and adding lots of interesting flavors to the meals on your plan. Even eating your meals and snacks has gone on auto-pilot and doesn't require nearly the attention and effort it once did.

This is good stuff, right? So why is it that you kind of feel like you're cheating or doing something wrong now that your new behaviors have transformed into healthy habits?

All of our lives, we've been programmed to think that weight-loss programs mean deprivation, starvation and misery.

And we've usually proven this to be true first-hand every time we've chosen to follow the latest fad diet. It only stands to reason that when you follow a healthy eating and exercise plan, and support it with mental and emotional resources, you may eventually get a little suspicious and wonder if your program is still working (even though you're not feeling deprived, starved and miserable).

Don't let the Mind play tricks on you!

You've been conditioned to associate certain feelings with a *weight-loss program* but here's where your association is missing the mark: did those feelings also correspond to *long-term weight-loss success*? I'm going to guess they didn't and that's why you're taking this journey again. So, my friend, although Deprivation, Starvation and Misery may have been your companions on previous weight-loss journeys, they weren't your allies and they didn't help you reach your final destination. It's not a good thing but a GREAT thing that you kicked them off the Weight Loss Wagon this time and took the journey without them. It's OK to think about them every once in a while but don't you dare think for one minute that you need to pick them up at the next station. A well-designed weight-loss program is created to work without those deadweights and you're doing just fine without them. Trust the process and keep on keeping on!

MINDSET TOOL:

If you're feeling as though your program is going too smoothly or that it's too easy and you want to increase the level of challenge simply to maintain your interest, don't focus on the food aspect. Look at your exercise program. Workout routines can easily be changed to increase intensity or variety or any number of other factors that will allow you to experience the level of challenge you desire without pushing you back into the deprivation, starvation and misery mindset. In fact, if you increase the intensity of your workouts considerably, you may need to adjust your meal plan and increase calories to keep up your energy levels.

DAY 24: Resistance, Acceptance, Change
MOOD INDICATOR: Feeling
resistant

A year and a half ago, my husband and I made the decision to get a puppy.

Well, let me rephrase that.

My husband talked me into getting – and keeping – a puppy. Frankly, I wasn't bought into the idea from the start and those who know me remember well that I did NOT embrace this new family member with open arms. In fact, I waged an all-out campaign to re-home her for at least the first four months that we had her. You see, while my husband was traveling for work at the time, I was left on my own trying to figure out how to train this little creature, who, by the way, wanted nothing to do with my structure, rules and discipline (imagine that!). And as much as the dog resisted me, I resisted her and we were constantly at odds with each other.

Fast forward a year and a half and this dog is now my shadow and best buddy. She follows me everywhere, snuggles beside me the moment she sees me sitting down (she's butted up against me in the armchair as I write this), and provides the unconditional love that every pet owner cherishes.

So what does any of this have to do with your weight-loss journey?

Weight loss and wellness are mental games. Being successful at managing your health requires the right mindset for adopting changes and making them last.

But change – in whatever form it may take – is something we humans are programmed to resist – even if the change is cute, fluffy and gives you wet kisses on the nose. If it's enough of a change and enough of a disruption to the status quo, the Mind automatically goes into resistance mode. So what then?

If you remember the game "Rock, Paper, Scissors," you likely remember that Rock beat Scissors, Scissors beat Paper, and Paper beat Rock. A similar game can be played when it comes to adopting new habits. I call it "Resistance, Acceptance, Change." The rules of the game are that Resistance beats Change, Change beats

Acceptance, Acceptance beats Resistance.

The secret to getting past the resistance stage is to first demonstrate acceptance of change. Acceptance overcomes resistance and paves the way for change and progress.

In order to build acceptance, you have to get on the same level as the change. Make friends with the change and challenge your fears about it. Figure out what the change is really all about. Study it like a research project. You may be surprised to find your fears and resistance melting in the wake of understanding and empathy and the change no longer feeling like the threat it once did.

In order for me to come to terms with the puppy, I had to accept that she was now part of the family and then get down on her level literally (playing with her on the floor, or "on her turf," so to speak) as well as figuratively (understanding her limitations as a puppy who had only been in this world a few short months). I also had to acknowledge my own fears about not knowing what the heck I was doing in terms of raising a dog (I mean, I had never even had a fish let alone a dog depend on me!). Accepting her enabled me to push past the resistance stage and develop a bond with her that has allowed us to reach a place I never could have imagined a year and a half ago.

MINDSET TOOL:

When we decide to adopt healthy habits but feel resistance (which happens even if we were the ones to initiate the new habits), it's important to get on the same level as the changes and face our fears head-on. Asking ourselves a series of "why" questions is often a useful tool for ferreting out the root cause of our worries and concerns and enabling us to regain control over them.

For example, if you decide to begin working out in a gym and purchase a membership but realize you're not going, ask yourself why.

The first answer may be, "I'm too busy."

So then ask, "Why are you too busy?"

"Because I work late every night and can't get up early in the morning to go."

"Why can't you get up in the morning and go?"

"Because I don't want to."

"Why don't you want to?"

"Because I don't think I am in good enough shape yet

to go to the gym."

And THERE YOU HAVE IT! Now you know the root cause and can address the issue at hand, which is not one of time or even desire but of poor body image. Knowing the root cause allows you to then channel your energy toward resolving the real issue so that you, too, can move past fear toward acceptance and ultimately make the change you set out to make.

Resistance and fear are powerful emotions and are inherent whenever you embark on a journey that involves change. It's important not to let these emotions paralyze you because such paralysis may prevent you from experiencing the surprising joy that change can bring, once you accept and embrace the change at hand.

DAY 25: It's an Invitation, Not an Obligation...Nor a Death Sentence!

MOOD INDICATOR: Feeling nervous about social obligations

It never fails. As soon as you start a weight-loss program, the deluge of invitations to parties and social gatherings begins. If you didn't know better, you'd think your friends and family picked up on the cosmic radar that you had hopped on the Weight Loss Wagon and that they were doing everything in their power to knock you off.

As if it's not enough that life in general has to go on despite the emotionally taxing journey on which you have embarked, every passenger on the Weight Loss Wagon must also contend with the possibility of being invited to social events that won't align with his/her meal plan. It's important to recognize from the start of your journey that this possibility is likely to happen, especially if your journey will take more than a month

or two. Birthdays creep up on the calendar, holidays
sneak in, and friends and family will inevitably find
one or more reasons to celebrate with food and drink at
some point during the course of your weight-loss
program.

The receipt of the ill-timed party invitation will likely
force you to feel a pit in your stomach and make your
brain race wildly as it desperately attempts to come up
with ways to either politely get out of attending the
event (and not feel guilty) or indulge in the event
without screwing up your progress and your entire
plan. God help you if the host or hostess is delivering
the invitation verbally because chances are that most of
the details will be lost in the ruckus of your mental
chatter.

**Though they require some careful handling,
social invitations are not the end of the world
when you're following a weight-loss program.
They, like everything else, simply require you to
have the right mindset.**

First, don't panic. While the social event is
undoubtedly important to the host/ess, bear in mind
that its importance is being exaggerated in your Mind
because of its potential impact on the success of your

weight-loss plan (which has become the focal point of your world over the past few days and weeks). Put this event into perspective relative to other things in your world (and even in the world of the host/ess) and you will soon realize that it may not be AS monumental as you first believed.

Second, even if the event is of significant importance, remember that the impact it bears on your weight-loss efforts is completely within your control. Neither the event nor the food at the event can control you, provided you don't give up the power that comes from having a plan and following it.

Finally, remove your ego from the equation. Though your presence at an event to which you are invited is obviously desired (hence the reason you were invited), it is highly unlikely that the event will be irreparably spoiled by your absence if you decide to opt out. There are some exceptions, of course, like the wedding of a child or other close relative, but for the average run-of-the-mill party invitation, this tends to be true. Checking your ego at the door enables you to gain even more perspective and accept your responsibility to do what is in your best interest to do.

MINDSET TOOL:

If you've received an invitation and followed the
guidelines above, you should now be calm and
collected and mentally able to make a sound decision
about your attendance at the event. If you're
wondering, "What decision? I can't say no!" you may
also wish to review the information for Day 19. "No" is
not only a legitimate answer but possibly the healthiest
answer you can give. If you are not comfortable in the
social setting you expect to find at a particular
event...if temptations will abound and you simply
haven't mastered the degree of discipline needed for
that kind of test...it is perfectly OK to recognize this
and to protect yourself from the situation. Graciously
explaining to your host/ess that you have embarked on
a weight-loss journey will likely be met with words of
encouragement and support. The reactions you fear
(insult or hurt feelings) are seldom what you
experience once the situation is explained.

If you would like to attend the event but aren't sure
you have the discipline required, find a quiet place
where you can be alone for a few minutes. Close your
eyes and visualize yourself attending the event.
Imagine yourself walking in. Picture your outfit and
how you look and feel. See yourself talking to other

guests and ultimately being confronted with the food and drink options. How do you feel then? What choices do you feel inclined to make? Play out the scenario for as long as possible and try to stay in every moment so that you have enough data to evaluate how you will likely respond in real life. Open your eyes and make an honest assessment. If you don't feel ready to take on the challenge of attending a social event, it may be too soon and it is probably in your best interest to decline for now.

If you decide that you're ready to tackle the festivities, it's important that you have a plan, whether the event is dinner at a restaurant or in a private home, or a full-blown party. Using the exercise described in the paragraph above will help even if you have no doubt about attending the event. By playing out the scenario in your Mind, you can put together a strategy for handling the details you may encounter. For small events like private dinner parties, you may need to explain to your host/ess your dietary limitations in advance so that they can either be accommodated or you can potentially bring your own food items to the event. Depending on how well you know the host/ess and your level of comfort, there are many creative options for approaching even the intimate affairs.

For larger parties, always plan to survey the buffet and

drink tables first. Do a complete walk-around. Never approach them with dish in hand, ready to load up on whatever grabs your attention. Remain mindful at all times and make conscious decisions that will fill you with nutritious vs. empty calories as much as possible. Once at an event, seek out others in similar situations. You may be able to bond with them and reinforce your commitment to have fun but not at the expense of your health and weight-loss program.

Being on a weight-loss journey doesn't mean you have to become a hermit and abstain from social events altogether. It does, however, mean that you have to follow an honest and mindful process for evaluating your readiness before committing to such events and then, for those to which you do commit, that you have a plan for handling yourself in each situation.

DAY 26: The Answer Is Never in the Refrigerator

MOOD INDICATOR: Feeling tempted to indulge in an emotional eating episode

You've now walked in and out of the kitchen for what may be the seventh or eighth time since you got home, each time pulling open the refrigerator door and peeking inside at least once per circuit.

So far so good though. You haven't gone past the peeking stage and, to anyone watching, you appear to be cool as a cucumber, going through the motions mechanically, much like a police officer walking his or her beat.

Little do these onlookers know the surge of emotions swamping you beneath the surface!

With each trip you make, the temptation to indulge in whatever delectables the refrigerator might hold becomes greater and greater. By the ninth or tenth round of duty, you're pretty sure you're destined to cave and have newfound appreciation for the reason why police officers flock to the local donut shops.

Stop the madness!!!

Obsessive kitchen and refrigerator tours don't qualify as your daily dose of physical activity!

There is something bigger going on here and the onus is on you, dear friend, to figure out what it is before it wins control over you. Often the obsessive repetition of behaviors like this signals boredom or anxiety (and sometimes anxiety's kindred spirit, procrastination). The Mind either lacks entertainment or is fretting over/dreading something. And because the Mind can be impatient when not given proper attention, it doesn't take long for the Mind to take charge and either entertain or distract itself because no one else is doing the job properly. It will literally begin to play games, especially with the Stomach, who is always an easy target to convince of things (like cravings) that aren't even close to being true. As the Stomach responds, the Mind gets the satisfaction of ending the boredom or creating a distraction from the anxiety. An emotional eating episode then ensues.

It's a cruel and twisted game but remember, our primal instincts are designed to protect us and, to that end, that's all the Mind is trying to do: "save us" from boredom and anxiety.

I am not going to get into the dynamics behind emotional eating in this book. For one, that's a much larger subject to which an entire book should be dedicated to do it justice – not just a single chapter. Secondly, the point of this chapter is not to understand those dynamics but to prevent them from happening in the first place. By recognizing the warning signs before emotional eating episodes occur, you will be better able to manage the situations in ways that help you avoid the emotional eating pitfall altogether.

MINDSET TOOL:

One warning sign of an oncoming emotional eating episode may be repetitive kitchen and refrigerator tours, as described above. If you find yourself falling into that kind of habit, even if you have not yet been lured into emotional eating, you need to nip it in the bud. The answer to whatever you are seeking is NOT in the refrigerator. I promise. But the truth is, you ARE seeking something. So what is it? If you're bored, what can you do to offset that boredom? Perhaps you can take a walk or call a friend or sit down and read a book or magazine in which you know you will become engrossed. Try to make the activity something that will take you away from the kitchen and get your Mind off food.

If you're anxious, what are you worrying about? Is there something you can do right now to offset some of that worry? If so, do it, or at least create an action plan to begin doing it. If it's a worry you can't address, consider why you're investing so much energy into it. Perhaps it's a serious concern, like the illness of a family member. That's certainly legitimate but also a worry over which you have no control. So perhaps the best thing to do with worries of that nature is to sit in meditation or prayer (if that's your preferred form of meditation) and spend time releasing the worry.

No matter what it is that is driving you toward the refrigerator door over and over and over again, I can assure you that there are ways to engage your Mind and address the root cause head-on. In doing so, you will create distraction and entertainment for your Mind and avert the temptation of emotional eating, which may otherwise sabotage your plans.

DAY 27: Failure vs. Setback

MOOD INDICATOR: Feeling like you need some slack

During the first 30 days of your weight-loss journey, when you're usually marching full-steam ahead and have laser-sharp focus on your weight-loss goals, it's easy to fall into the trap of an "all or nothing mentality."

You have days when you are spot-on with your program and you nail it. No deviations from your eating plan or your workouts. You're strutting around like a proud peacock, thinking you're truly da bomb!

And then you have days when you're hanging your head low, beating yourself up for what your overachieving Mind considers to be cataclysmic slip-ups.

Your weight-loss goal doesn't have an expiration date.

Sure, you may have a target date by which you want to hit your goal and there is no question that the sooner you can adopt healthier habits the better it will be for your overall wellness, but in reality, there is no hard and fast date by which you MUST lose weight (barring weight loss that may be required for medical/surgical reasons, but in the interest of the average reader, I am going to assume that your program does not fall in that category). The pressure you feel when you have a "bad" day and think all hope for achieving your goals is lost because you ate that forbidden cookie or skipped your workout for two days in a row is entirely self-imposed. While this type of pressure can be motivational at times, it can also have the opposite effect when you don't cut yourself any slack, and it's important for you to understand where the line should be drawn.

MINDSET TOOL:

The next time you feel panicky that something you ate or did (or didn't eat or didn't do) is going to sabotage your entire weight-loss journey, take a moment to just breeeeeeeeeeeeathe.

I mean that literally (yep, sometimes it's that easy!).

One long breath can do wonders for clearing the Mind and regaining perspective.

Now that you're thinking clearly again, look at the incident in terms of the big picture. One deviation is not going to erase all of your progress (and if you've been reading this book and using its tools, you ought to be experiencing such deviations in isolation and correcting them as they occur – not ignoring them and allowing them to pick up steam like a snowball rolling down a mountain, becoming an avalanche of deviations before you even realize it). Depending on the nature of the deviation, it may set you back a little bit and you may want to work a little harder or tighten up your program in other ways to offset the setback and get back on the original timeline to meet your goals. After you take that deep breath, evaluate how much of an impact your deviation may really have on your plan and what you want to do next. If you're working with a professional, consider picking up the phone or writing an email for his/her opinion. If you're working alone, go online and (if you don't already follow them) find some weight-loss groups on Facebook and join them. Social media can provide free support and is a great platform for posting questions to find out how others have dealt with similar situations.

It's also important to view each deviation or lapse in judgment as a lesson to be learned. After you've got things back under control, reflect on the deviation and ask yourself some hard questions about why you were tempted to deviate. Is your plan too strict? Were you acting on emotional impulses and trying to hide your feelings behind food? What was the trigger? Sometimes eating one food can trigger your uncontrolled desire for another (for example, chewing sugar-free gum is used by many people to curb an interest in eating but for other people, the sugar alcohols in gum can trigger sugar cravings so strong that the minute the gum has been spit out, these people find themselves reaching for the first sugar-laden item they can find).

Sometimes a series of seemingly harmless decisions set you up for a lapse or deviation. For instance, buying foods not included on your eating plan "in case guests come over" creates conditions that can easily lead to a lapse in judgment.

Use every slip-up, every lapse, every deviation as an opportunity to better understand yourself and potentially tweak your program to better work for you.

And as I mentioned earlier, never forget that YOU own your weight-loss timeline. You can set your goals to be met whenever you want to meet them. It's great to be aggressive and grab the bull by the horns, but if you need to make adjustments along the way, that's OK, too. It does NOT make you a failure. A failure is not someone who has a slip-up or experiences a setback. A failure is someone who stops trying altogether…and since you're still reading this book and pushing through the mental obstacles that every rider of the Weight Loss Wagon faces, I can assure you – you are no failure!

DAY 28: The Power of Words

**MOOD INDICATOR: Stable and
clear but always looking for ways to
fine-tune things**

Not long ago, a friend and I were talking about
Americans' seeming addiction to weight-loss
programs. During our conversation, he made the
observation that in India, where he had lived for some
period of time, people do not talk about losing weight
because "losing" implies they have an intention of
replacing it. Instead, they talk about "reducing."

How simple and yet...how brilliant!

The power of words is a theme often used in
motivational/inspirational quotes and is advocated by
circles that teach the benefits of positive thinking.
Many religions also make reference to the power of
words in their teachings.

Ironically, despite all the attention given to words and

the influence they may have, we still often miss the point. Perhaps because of all the mainstream chatter about words, many of us have diluted their power down to this: "say kind things and think positive thoughts." Why? Well…because it's what you've heard you should do to be happy. And it's trendy. And who doesn't want to be happy and trendy?

Embracing the ideas of "saying kind things" and "thinking positive thoughts" is a step in the right direction but the real lesson to learn is that ALL words have power, not just words strung together into sentences that express our opinions about other people, ourselves or a situation.

Think about that for a second.

Every single word has power of its own. Sometimes this power is primal and comes from somewhere deep inside of us that we may not even be able to explain. For example, say the word "disgust" and what do you feel? Most of us will feel a twinge in our stomach and perhaps even a physical withdrawal or a scrunch of the nose. But when you change that word to "disappointment," you're likely to have a softened response and may even feel sadness.

So what does all this mean for you on your weight-loss

journey?

Obviously, you can't be expected to walk around weighing every single word before it passes your lips but you may be able to use the power of words to help you navigate rough waters, avoid weight-loss pitfalls, or give yourself an extra boost of motivation when needed.

MINDSET TOOL:

Although words can't change reality, they can shape our perception of reality…and sometimes that's enough. Merely changing our perception may be all we need to push past an obstacle, confront a challenge, or simply keep ourselves on course.

Think about some of the words you use most often. In general, are they uplifting and encouraging or are they negative and discouraging? What about the ones you use relative to whatever obstacle or challenge you are facing? For example, let's say your family is not supportive of your weight-loss journey and keeps leaving snack food out on the counter or bringing home fast food or ordering pizza. It's easy to become resentful and angry and to begin to dread coming home to face these temptations. You may begin to feel depressed and beaten, knowing that you can only withstand the temptations for so long. You not only cuss out your family members in your head but have begun to have verbal arguments with them about their behavior.

None of this is helping you on your weight-loss journey and since your family is unlikely to change their behaviors for you (given that they haven't yet done so), it's up to you to reframe reality with the words you choose to associate with their actions. This will need to be done on the mental as well as verbal plane. Your thoughts about your family members' behaviors will need to transform from angry, resentful ones into forgiving and tolerant ones that accept their limitations to understand the journey you are taking. The words you verbally use to address them about their behaviors will need to transform from words of frustration and despair into ones that also reflect acceptance. It is only through acceptance that you will be able to find a place of inner calm where you can think clearly and tap into your resolve and discipline to follow your program despite the obstacles your family presents.

If your obstacles come in the form of your inner dialogue and the things you say to yourself, think about all of the words you use that bring you down emotionally, however slightly. This can include your use of the term "weight loss" (which may imply deprivation/restriction and have a negative connotation for you) and you may decide you want to follow the practice used in India and refer to it as "weight reduction" or simply "reducing" – whatever suits you! I personally refuse to use the word "diet" because it has so many negative connotations for me (not to mention that it includes the word "die"). Eliminating that word from my vocabulary and replacing it with the terms "healthy eating habits" and "healthy meal plans" puts my focus on the positive and what I am gaining (health!) vs. the limitations to which I am subjecting myself.

As simple and insignificant as words may seem, they possess incredible power. By using them to your advantage, you're adding one more resource to your weight-loss toolkit and improving the odds of your success.

DAY 29: Relapse Prevention Planning

MOOD INDICATOR: Feeling optimistic but realistic about the future and its challenges

"It's not difficult to stop smoking; I've done it dozens of times." ~ Mark Twain

This book is about reality.

And being human.

And part of reality and being human means that no matter how well you're doing on your weight-loss journey right now…and no matter how well you vow to do for the remainder of your program and beyond…you need to have a Relapse Prevention Plan.

By thinking ahead, and by working out ways to handle the temptation to slip back into "less healthy" habits, you can approach every step of your journey, as well as your life beyond your weight-loss program, with a greater sense of confidence.

Preparation breeds confidence and confidence breeds success.

You may never need to implement your Relapse Prevention Plan but knowing that you have one does wonders for your self-assurance.

I'm not saying you need to have a strict plan mapped out regarding the food you will/will not eat or how many drinks you will/will not have every day for the rest of your life. That's completely unrealistic and that's not what Relapse Prevention Planning is about. When I talk about creating a Relapse Prevention Plan, I'm asking you to focus on your ability to handle high-risk situations and cope with temptation.

MINDSET TOOL:

First, identify things you would consider "high-risk situations." For many of us, these are social events like birthday parties, holiday gatherings, work functions, etc. – events at which you may feel peer pressure to eat and drink like everyone else (vs. eating and drinking in ways you know your body can tolerate) and especially ones at which you aren't surrounded by close friends and family members with whom you may feel more comfortable explaining your limitations. For those of us whose family members happen to be the least supportive of our efforts, high-risk situations may include extended family gatherings or, in the absolute worst-case scenario, daily dinners with immediate family.

Whatever situations make you feel the most pressure to deviate from the healthy habits you have been practicing, THOSE are your high-risk situations. List them out on a sheet of paper then, beside each one, jot down coping skills you can use to manage each situation. For example, if attending a party has the potential to derail your healthy eating habits, you may want to eat a small, healthy meal before attending so that hunger pains won't attack and convince you to make poor food choices on impulse. Or maybe you do that and make a written contract with yourself to drink a glass of water – a full, 8-ounce glass (none of this sippy cup stuff!) – before you allow yourself to have a glass of wine. By alternating water and alcohol in your hands, you're less likely to consume quite as many calories as you would otherwise consume, and by putting that contract with yourself in writing, you have a more formal commitment by which you may feel obligated to stand.

Be creative when thinking of ways to cope and don't forget to use the visualization tool to help you as well (see Day 21). Playing out scenarios in your head in vivid detail often sparks new ideas for coping and gets you more fully prepared once the actual situation plays out.

Relapse Prevention Planning is planning for success when it comes to sustainable weight loss and lifelong wellness.

Though you may have dismissed my opening quote from Mark Twain as mere humor and think that Relapse Prevention Planning is a tool you really don't need, I hope you trust me when I say that a relapse can catch you unawares and that being proactive in thinking about your approach will be time well spent.

DAY 30: Setting Other Goals

MOOD INDICATOR: Feeling victorious and happy

Drum roll, please!!!

You did it! You just completed 30 days of your weight-loss program and that deserves a high five, fist bump AND a 21-gun salute!

For a handful of you, this may be the end of your journey. Thirty days was all you set out to do and you accomplished what you wanted to achieve within that timeframe.

For most of you, this is only the beginning. Your weight-loss journey will likely continue for another 30, 60 or 90+ days and will probably include various stages as you transition from the most restrictive phase at the beginning to the more liberal maintenance eating phase at the end of the program. The temptation to celebrate your success right now will be strong – and hopefully you DO have some sort of celebration built into your plan – but the reality is that there's more hard work ahead for you.

Throughout the remaining days of your weight-loss journey, you will likely ride a roller coaster of emotions similar to the one you rode during the first 30 days. The information contained in this book can be leveraged throughout your trip and can be applied at any time. For instance, there are definitely going to be days when you get frustrated with your family and friends or don't know how to handle an invitation to a party at which you know culinary temptations will abound. Don't be afraid to crack open this book and use the relevant chapters as reminders for how to navigate through rough waters. And just because you read a chapter once doesn't necessarily mean you internalized all of its messages. Upon your second or third or even fourth reading, you may very well discover new messages or things you overlooked the first few times around.

MINDSET TOOL:

As a final tool I'd like to offer you for the remainder of your journey, or even if you're journey has now ended, consider setting a goal for the next 30 days that has absolutely nothing to do with weight loss.

It doesn't have to be big. It can be as simple as setting a goal to clean out your closet or a room in your house (or even just a drawer) that has become a "dumping ground" (removing clutter in our environment almost always helps us mentally and emotionally and lowers stress levels). Or it can be something like committing to go somewhere you've wanted to go but have put off doing. Or carving out time to spend with someone you may have been neglecting or time to read a book. The possibilities are endless and it's entirely up to you to select the goal. However, by focusing on things other than the specific elements of your weight-loss plan (i.e., the food, the meal planning, the workouts, etc.), you decrease the risk of burnout and of turning what has thus far been a positive experience into a chore. And what's great is that setting and working toward these other goals actually promotes balance…and balance supports a greater sense of overall well-being.

You're setting the stage for a lifetime of healthy habits, balance and harmony.

What better way to approach the next segment of your journey and the rest of your life?

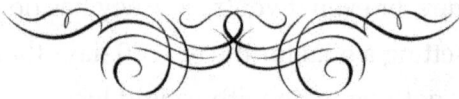

About the Author

Dale Barr is a 20-year veteran of leading process and behavioral change initiatives in corporate America and is a survivor of the multisensory overload and consequent wellness burnout experienced by many business professionals.

Dale's passion for health and wellness began at a very young age, reinforced by her involvement in competitive gymnastics and a mother who used holistic health strategies long before doing so was trendy. After competing in and winning her first National Physique Committee (NPC) figure competition at the age of 40, and then contending with some of her own health challenges shortly after, Dale was inspired to use her passion to help others master the wellness mindset and reach their wellness goals. Upon earning certifications in health and wellness coaching, wellness and nutrition consulting, personal training, and herbalism, she founded Wellness Rehab, LLC – an online wellness coaching service that helps clients make sustainable lifestyle changes and find more balanced states of well-being.

* 9 7 8 0 9 8 9 9 9 4 8 6 0 9 *